Van Dyck in Sicily

Xavier F. Salomon

Van Dyck in Sicily
1624 - 1625 Painting and the Plague

Dulwich Picture Gallery, London

SilvanaEditoriale

Cover illustration
Emanuele Filiberto of Savoy, detail (cat. 2)

Silvana Editoriale

Produced by
Arti Grafiche Amilcare Pizzi Spa

Direction
Dario Cimorelli

Art Director
Giacomo Merli

Copy Editor
Paola Rossi

Layout
Annamaria Ardizzi

Production Coordinator
Michela Bramati

Editorial Assistant
Emma Altomare

Iconographic Office
Alessandra Olivari, Michela Pittaluga

Press Office
Lidia Masolini, press@silvanaeditoriale.it

First published to accompany the exhibition

VAN DYCK IN SICILY
1624 - 1625 PAINTING AND THE PLAGUE

Dulwich Picture Gallery
Gallery Road, London, SE21 7AD

15 February – 27 May 2012

DULWICH PICTURE GALLERY
REDISCOVERING OLD MASTERS: THE MELOSI SERIES

FRIENDS OF DULWICH PICTURE GALLERY

AMERICAN FRIENDS OF
DULWICH PICTURE GALLERY

The grant from the American Friends of Dulwich Picture Gallery Inc. was made possible through the generosity of The Arthur and Holly Magill Foundation.

Xavier F. Salomon
Curator of Southern Baroque, Department of European Paintings, The Metropolitan Museum of Art, New York

Ian A.C. Dejardin
Director

Xavier Bray
Arturo and Holly Melosi Chief Curator

Exhibitions
Clare Simpson
Philippa Hemsley
Assisted by Rebecca England

Catalogue Copy Editors
Julie Pickard
Paola Rossi

Development and Communications
Lily Harriss
Julia Lindon
James Thompson

Press and Marketing
Ellie Manwell
Madeline Adeane
Andrea Szeplaki

This exhibition has been made possible with the assistance of the Government Indemnity Scheme, which is provided by the Department for Culture, Media and Sport, administered by the Arts Council England.

The Melosi Series at Dulwich Picture Gallery has become one of the gallery's most significant strands of exhibitions, devoted to Old Masters and – through the enlightened interest of the American Friends of Dulwich Picture Gallery, supported through the generosity of The Arthur and Holly Magill Foundation and Arturo and Holly Melosi – often focusing on facets of art history that might otherwise be overlooked.

Sir Anthony van Dyck, at first glance, might therefore seem an unlikely subject, simply through being so famous and so well-served by exhibitions. We all know and love the swagger portraits. However, Dr Xavier Salomon, until 2010 the Arturo and Holly Melosi Chief Curator here at Dulwich, was inspired by Dulwich's own great portrait by Van Dyck of Emanuele Filiberto, the Viceroy of Sicily, and has uncovered a fascinating story that makes it a natural 'Melosi show'. The year and a half that Van Dyck spent on the island turns out to have been something of a turning point in the young artist's career. The blood turns cold at how close he must have been to suffering the same fate as his illustrious sitter, when the outbreak of plague effectively marooned him in Palermo. In fact, in some ways he was in the right place at the right time, because the discovery of the relics of Saint Rosalia, and the religious fervour that greeted it, gave him the opportunity to establish the Saint's visual iconography and produce several versions. Similarly, he was just in time to meet a legend, the extremely elderly portraitist Sofonisba Anguissola, and record the meeting in his diary – and what a meeting that must have been, between the ancient aristocrat and the young prince of the brush, Van Dyck, with the plumes in his hat and his gold bling. Dr Salomon has painted us a profound and scholarly portrait himself: of an artist, a patron and a city brought together at a critical moment. Emanuele Filiberto didn't survive the plague, but he was fortunate in his young portraitist – the viceroy's face, and that astonishing armour which will be on display beside the portrait, will never be forgotten.

The exhibition could not have happened without the American Friends of Dulwich Picture Gallery and Arturo and Holly Melosi's impassioned interest and support; my deepest gratitude to them. And as always, we have been able to rely on the dedicated support of the Friends of Dulwich Picture Gallery. Philippa Hemsley, Exhibitions Officer, took on the administration of the exhibition, succeeding Emily Goalen in that role, under the watchful eye of Sarah Clarke, Head of Exhibitions, who was herself succeeded by Clare Simpson. Finally, my thanks and congratulations must go to my former colleague, Xavier Salomon, who committed to deliver this very personal project despite his move to a prestigious new job at The Metropolitan Museum of Art in New York.

Ian A.C. Dejardin
The Sackler Director

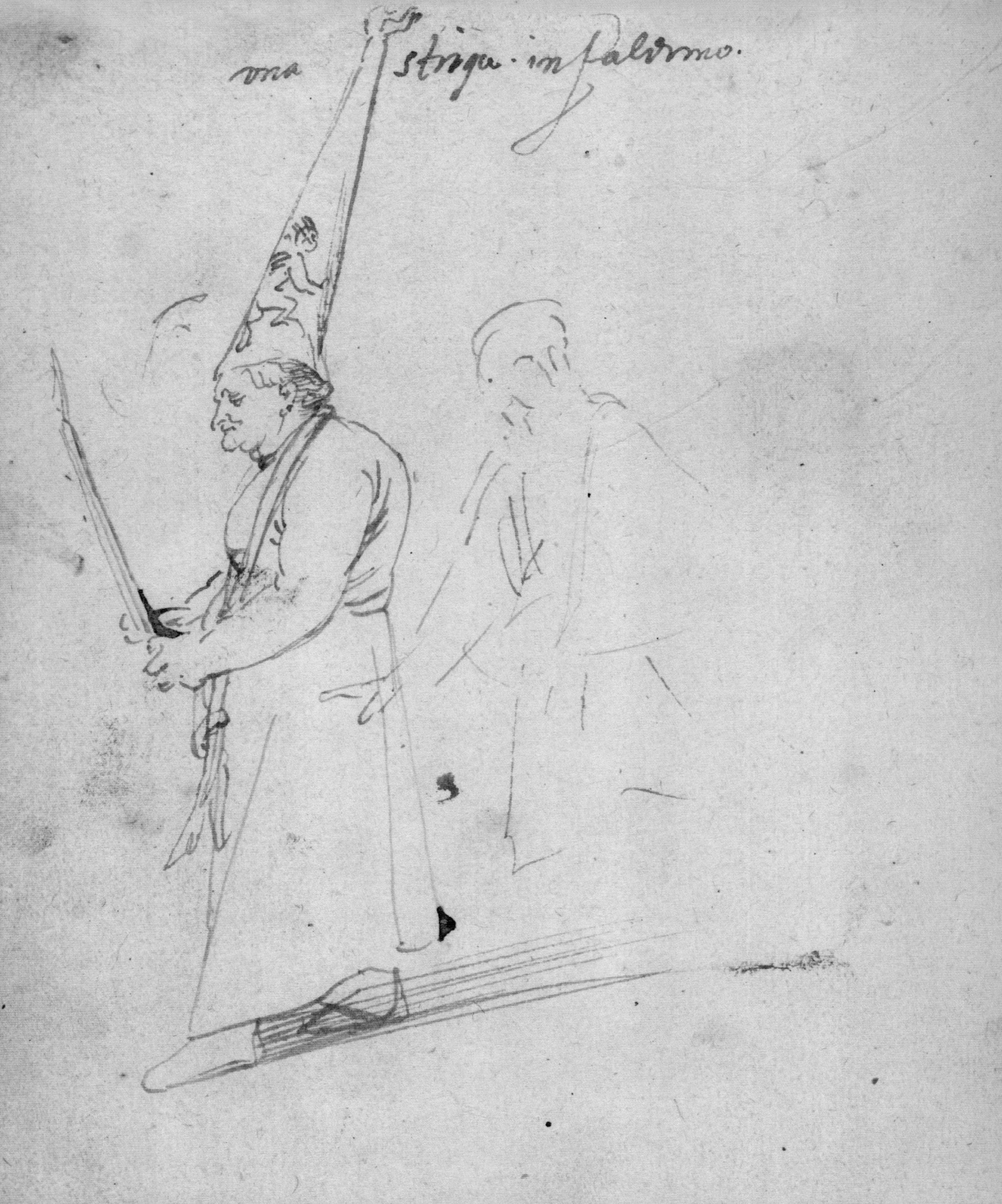
vna striga · in palermo ·

Contents

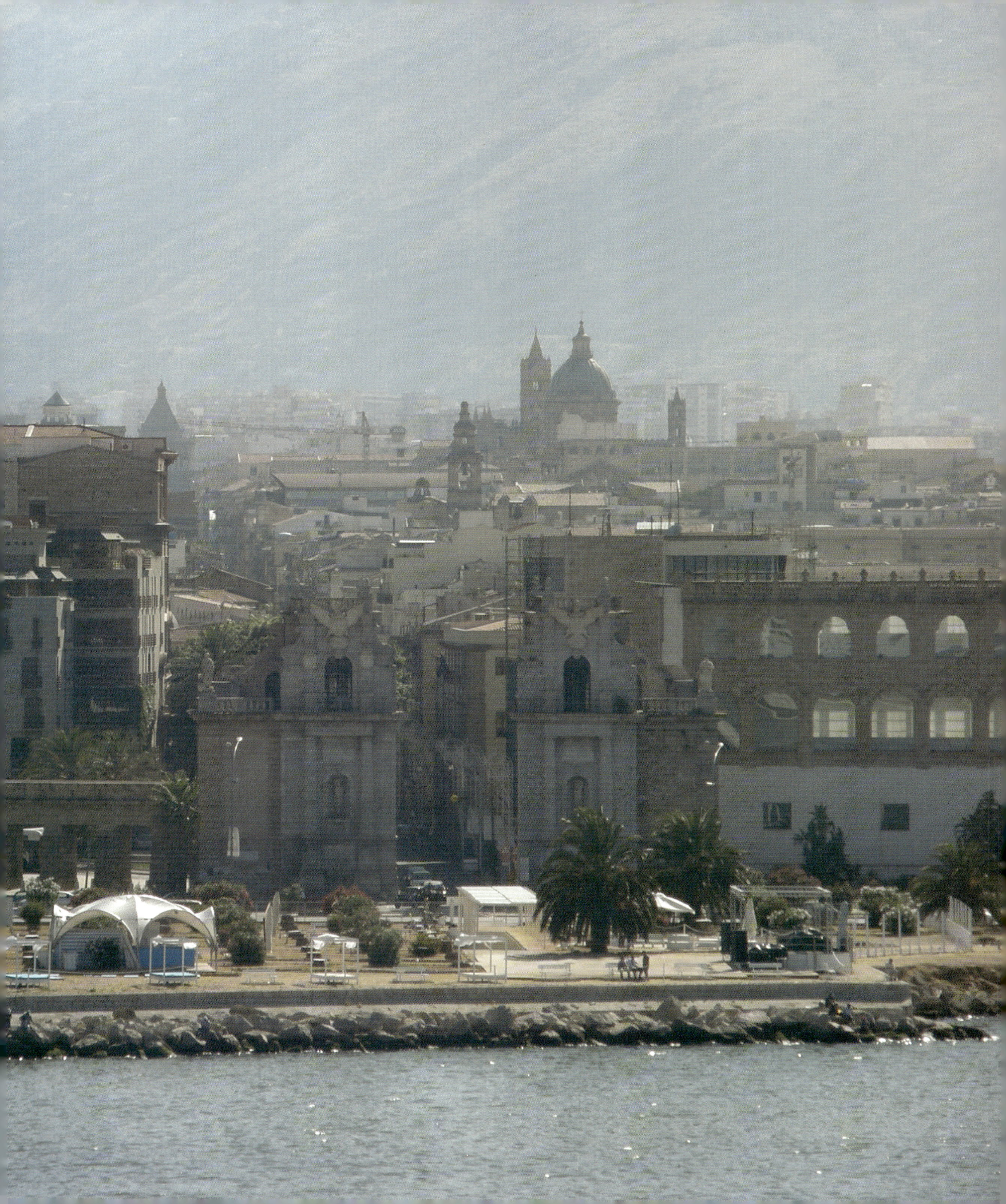

Introduction

Xavier F. Salomon

In the spring of 1624, the twenty-five-year-old Anthony van Dyck boarded a ship in the harbour of Genoa. He had lived in Italy already for almost three years, having moved from Antwerp. The boat was to carry the young Flemish painter along the Tyrrhenian coast of the Mediterranean Sea, pausing briefly at the harbours of Portovenere, Leghorn, Piombino, Porto Ercole, Foce del Tevere, Nettuno, Gaeta, Pozzuoli, Naples, Camerota, Diamante and Messina. The destination was Palermo, capital of Sicily, governed at the time by a Spanish viceroy. It was the viceroy himself who had invited Van Dyck to his capital with the prestigious commission to paint his portrait. The artist immortalised Emanuele Filiberto of Savoy that spring, soon after his arrival in Palermo. The viceroy was shown by Van Dyck in his armour, resplendent in black and gold and emblazoned with the Savoy emblems of knots, crowns and palm trees. With the death of the sitter, only a few months later, the armour and the portrait were dispersed, one headed to Madrid and the king's armoury, the other probably to the court of the viceroy's father, in Turin. The portrait is now at Dulwich Picture Gallery, the armour still in the Real Armería in Madrid. This exhibition has its roots in the idea of reuniting the sitter and his armour in a temporary display. While this project started to take shape, the armour and the portrait were shown together twice in large exhibitions, one dedicated to the Savoy dynasty, in the palace at Venaria Reale, in the outskirts of Turin, in 2007, the other focusing on armours from the Real Armería and their representations in paintings, at the National Gallery of Art in Washington, in 2009.

The plan to bring together the sitter and his armour in London soon expanded into a broader exhibition. Van Dyck arrived in Sicily at a difficult time; a few months after the ship that brought him to the island moored in Palermo, the bubonic plague hit the city. Emanuele Filiberto was the pestilence's most prominent victim. Until recently, it was believed that Van Dyck had managed to escape from Sicily only a few months after, in 1624. However, recent research carried out by an Italian scholar, Giovanni Mendola, has revealed that the painter stayed in Palermo longer than expected, until the autumn of 1625. During the year and a half of his residence in Palermo, Van Dyck lived through one of the most violent epidemics of seventeenth-century Italy. It is worth contemplating what difference Van Dyck's death in Palermo would have made to the history of art – how different the course of English portraiture would have been, for example, without Van Dyck ever having lived for ten years at the court of King Charles I, between 1632 and 1641. Yet Van Dyck survived the plague in an almost miraculous fashion, unscathed by the disease that killed tens of thousands of people in Palermo alone. What the artist did during these terrifying months is still little known, notwithstanding the survival of archival documents that give us a glimpse of commissions, rental payments and other financial transactions that Van Dyck was involved with. The studies of Mendola and of Vincenzo Abbate in the context of Van Dyck's Sicilian period are fundamental in understanding the broader picture of this phase in the artist's life.

Almost four hundred years after Van Dyck's journey, I decided to follow in his footsteps, and in July 2010 embarked on a very different ship from Genoa to Palermo. The city I left behind and the one I reached have changed significantly since Van Dyck was there, but trying to follow the painter, the places he might have known and seen, demonstrated how Genoa and Palermo have remained fundamentally close to their seventeenth-century counterparts, compared with many other cities in Europe. The house where Van Dyck lived in Palermo is long gone, replaced by modern buildings (fig. 9), but the Strada del Cassaro, the harbour of La Cala, the church of Santa Maria di Portosalvo are still there, giving a glimpse of Van Dyck's surroundings in 1624–25. As many of the palaces of the Genoese aristocracy that Van Dyck would have known well still survive on the Strada Nuova, so Emanuele Filiberto's Royal Palace

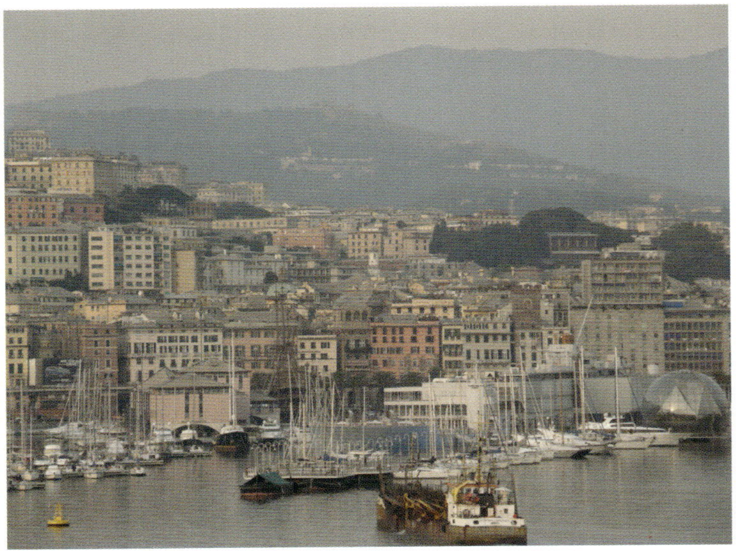

Genoa

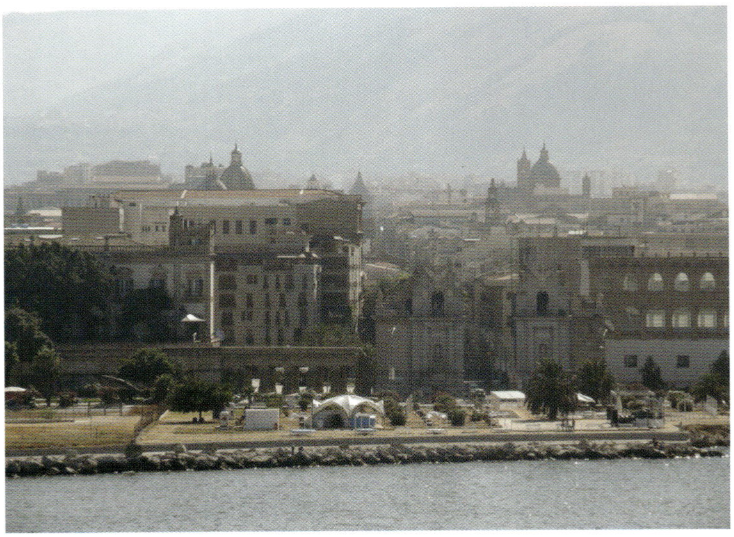

Palermo

is effectively similar to how Van Dyck would have known it. My Sicilian summer of research brought me to the libraries and archives of Palermo, following the trail inspiringly laid out by Abbate and Mendola, looking again at documents that provide the information we have on Van Dyck's period in Palermo. The figure of Emanuele Filiberto of Savoy, in particular, recently studied in detail by Maria Beatrice Failla, was fundamental for my research and for understanding Van Dyck's reason to travel to Sicily. But other characters also emerged as having been particularly important for Van Dyck in Palermo: the ruthless Archbishop Giannettino Doria, the Flemish Consul (and possibly a relative of the painter) Hendrik Dych, the elderly female painter Sofonisba Anguissola and her husband Orazio Lomellini, the Genoese merchant Desiderio Segno, the collector, dealer and thief Fabrizio Valguarnera, and a series of other artists, collectors and personalities in the city. Piecing the surviving information together tells a fascinating story. This exhibition catalogue brings together the threads of the research of many scholars on some of these individuals, in trying to give a complete – as much as possible – picture of Van Dyck's stay in Sicily.

The exhibition reunites for the first time all of the works that are documented, or believed to have been painted, between 1624 and 1625 in Palermo. They are portraits (cats. 2, 5, 6, 8) and paintings of religious subjects (cats. 9–10). The only work by Van Dyck still in Sicily, the *Madonna of the Rosary* in the Oratorio del SS. Rosario at San Domenico (fig. 33), is the only one not in the present exhibition. Even though it was commissioned in Palermo and intended for the oratory, it was painted entirely in Genoa, after Van Dyck left Sicily, between 1625 and 1628. The most significant group of paintings produced by Van Dyck in Palermo are the images of the city's patron saint, Rosalia (cats. 12–16). The relationship between the *santuzza* and her city has its roots in the summer of 1624, when her relics were found, processed through the city, and her name was on everybody's lips in the hope that she could vanquish the plague through her celestial intercession. Not only did Van Dyck create Rosalia's iconography as we know it today, but he also witnessed the events of that summer that fixed the saint's role for the city. He must have been present at the first *festino* in July 1625, and experiencing the same event hundreds of years later, in July 2010, makes one realise how deep and life changing the finding of the saint's relics has been for Palermo. The saint is still to this day highly venerated by the citizens of Palermo, to the point that the uniform of the city's football team is Rosalia's colour, pink. Van Dyck's fundamental role in shaping the image of Saint Rosalia has been fully explored by Gauvin Alexander Bailey in a fascinating essay in the catalogue for the 2005 exhibition *Hope and Healing. Painting in Italy in a Time of Plague 1500–1800* at the Worcester Art Museum in Massachusetts. The two paintings of Rosalia by Van Dyck in North American collections, from Houston (cat. 14) and New York (cat. 16), were brought together for that show. The present exhibition brings together every painting of Rosalia by Van Dyck, not only

Feast of Saint Rosalia, Palermo

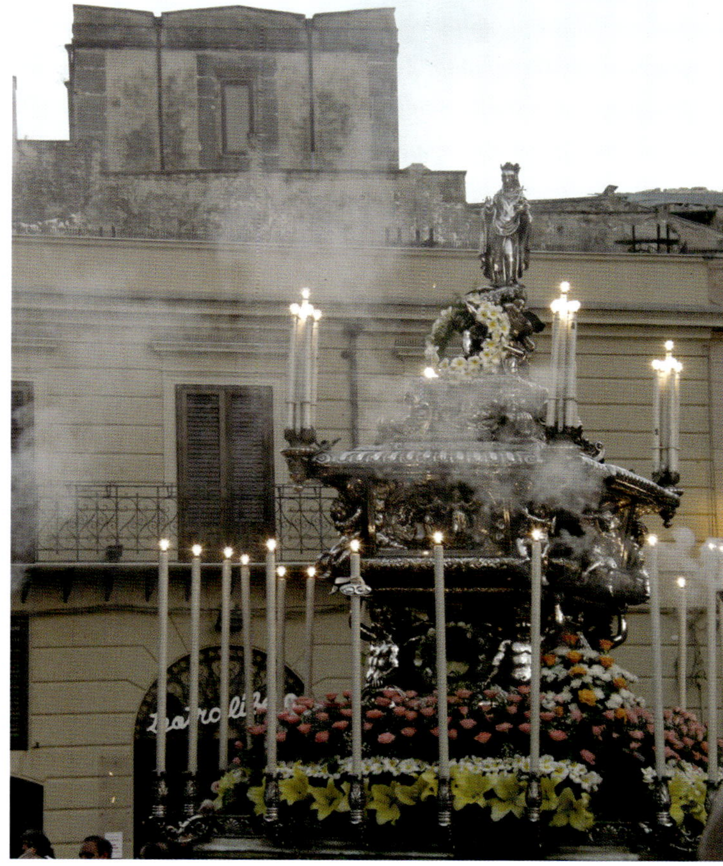

from America, but also from London (cat. 13), Spain (cat. 15) and Puerto Rico (cat. 12), allowing for them to be seen in the same room for the first time.

In writing this catalogue, the scholarly work of Vincenzo Abbate, Gauvin Alexander Bailey, Maria Beatrice Failla and Giovanni Mendola has supplied the foundations on which my research rests. Without their contributions, Charles Sterling's statement in 1939 that 'there is a period in Van Dyck's career of which extremely little is known and that is the time of his stay in Palermo' would still hold true. My greatest acknowledgement is therefore to them. Special thanks also goes to Susan Barnes and Piero Boccardo, the foremost experts on Van Dyck's Italian years, who have helped me along the way with this exhibition, from locations as far away as Genoa and Austin, Texas. Many friends and colleagues have been invaluable during the last five years and have contributed in many ways to my work on this exhibition, between London and New York, Genoa and Palermo. In particular I would like to thank Stijn Alsteens, Luigi Berio, Jonathan Bober, Edgar Peters Bowron, Xavier Bray, Dirk Breiding, Duncan Bull, Hugo Chapman, Keith Christiansen, Sarah Clarke, Michael Roque Collins, Nicholas Cullinan, Clare Elliott, Everett Fahy, Gabriele Finaldi, Michael Gallagher, Emily Goalen, Charlotte Hale, Harry Hancock, Cheryl Hartup, Philippa Hemsley, Elisabeth Hipp, Andrea Illescas, Lauren Jacobi, David Jaffè, Susan Jenkins, Alastair Laing, Walter Liedtke, Sara Mittica, Sarah Moulden, Robert Oresko (†), Pierfrancesco Palazzotto, Pablo Perez d'Ors, Kevin Petkos, Sophie Plender, Stuart Pyhrr, Valentina Ravaglia, Martin Royalton-Kisch, Francis Russell, Nicole Ryder, Mella Shaw, Nat Silver, Clare Simpson, Álvaro Soler del Campo, Luke Syson, Emanuela Tarizzo, Ian Thompson, An Van Camp, Alejandro Vergara and Robert Wald.

I would like to dedicate this exhibition and catalogue to my brother, Thomas Clement Salomon.

Van Dyck in Sicily

Xavier F. Salomon

'At the front, the ornately vested priest walked to and fro, doing his business and chanting. Incense billowed up, clouding the feeble flames of the altar candles, and with its heavy, sweet sacrificial odour another seemed to mingle: the smell of the sick city.'
Thomas Mann

The twenty-three-year-old Anthony van Dyck reached Rome, for the first time, in the early months of 1622. Giovan Pietro Bellori, in his 1672 biography of the painter, provided a vivid portrayal of him: 'he was still young, his beard barely sprouting, yet his youth was accompanied by grave modesty of character and nobility of mien, albeit he was small in stature. His manners were those of a lord rather than a commoner, and he appeared resplendent in rich attire of suits and court dress, because he had been accustomed to the society of noblemen in the school of Rubens; and being by nature grand and eager to become famous, therefore, in addition to his fine clothes, he adorned his head with plumes and hatbands, wore gold chains crossed on his chest, and kept a retinue of servants.'[1] Van Dyck's *Self-Portraits* from these years (fig. 1 and cat. 1) are a visual parallel to Bellori's text, and give us the image of a dashing young artist presenting himself to his public as a man of aristocratic and refined taste. Having left Antwerp, his birthplace, for a brief period in England, where he spent four months, between November 1620 and February 1621, at the court of King James I, Van Dyck moved to Italy in the early 1620s and lived there for six years. On 3 October 1621 he left Antwerp for Genoa, where he arrived by 20 November.[2] Waiting for him in the city were his two Flemish friends, Lucas and Cornelis de Wael (fig. 2). Nephews of Jan Brueghel the Elder, the De Wael brothers had established themselves in Genoa in the early 1620s, and together with the painter Jan Roos had become pillars of the Flemish artistic community in the city. They were to remain a firm point in Van Dyck's Italian years, and his double portrait of 1627 is a testament to such close friendship.[3] It was said that Cornelis was 'so generous that his house was always open to everyone and especially to his fellow-countrymen', and Van Dyck stayed with the brothers at their houses by Porta Santa Caterina all'Acquasola and near the Convent of Santa Brigida.[4]

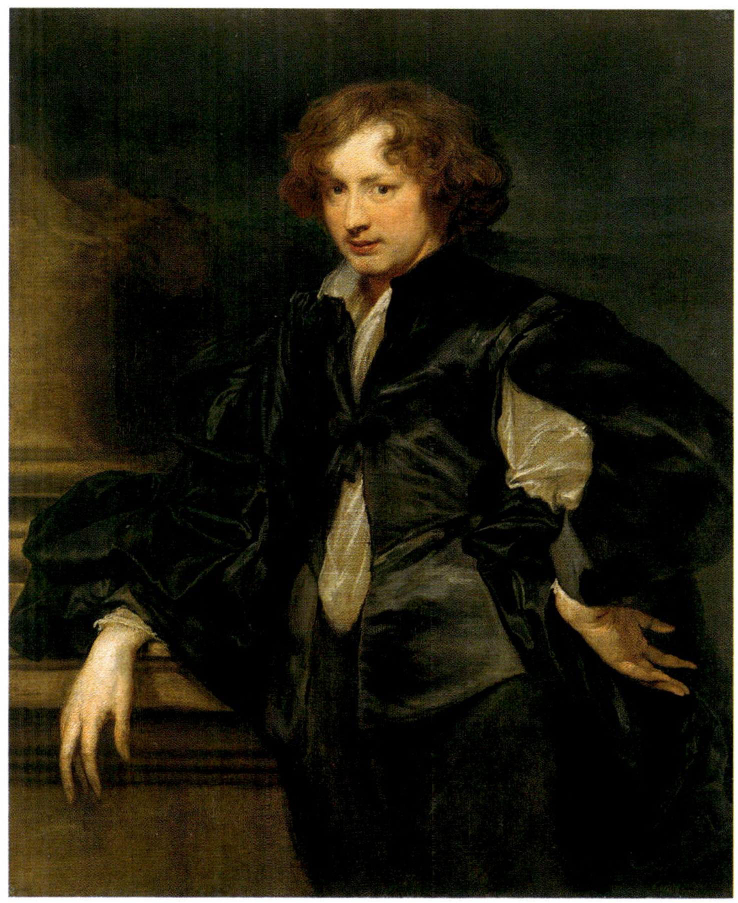

1 | Sir Anthony van Dyck, *Self-Portrait*
The State Hermitage Museum, Saint Petersburg

Van Dyck's choice to move to Italy was most likely due to his close relationship with Peter Paul Rubens, and his period as his

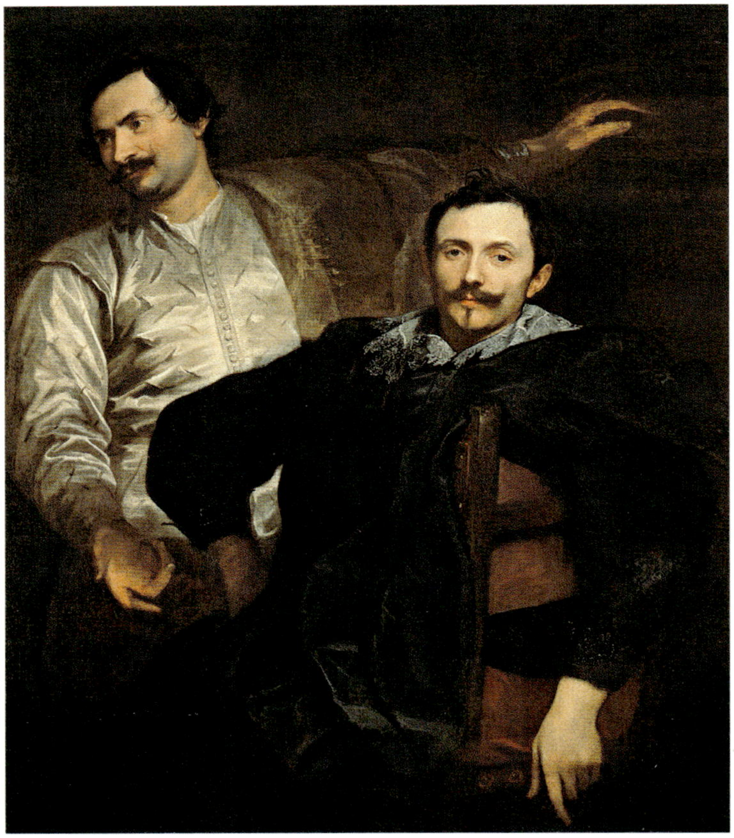

2 | Sir Anthony van Dyck,
Lucas and Cornelis de Wael
Pinacoteca Capitolina, Rome

3 | Sir Anthony van Dyck,
Cardinal Guido Bentivoglio
Palazzo Pitti, Florence

student in Antwerp. Rubens himself had lived in Italy for eight years, twenty years before, and had links with many Italian aristocratic families. It is, therefore, not surprising that the young Van Dyck would have chosen to follow in Rubens's footsteps and ventured south to Italy, where he could have studied antiquities and the works of Old Masters. His small sketchbook (figs. 6–8, 21 and cat. 5) demonstrates the range of artworks that Van Dyck studied during his Italian sojourn. While the harbour city of Genoa was to remain the painter's main base in Italy, he also travelled extensively. By February 1622 he was in Rome, where he stayed until August; this was followed by a visit of a few months to Venice before returning to Rome in early 1623. He may have visited Turin and Florence on his way south, and remained in the papal city for eight months. By late 1623 he was back in Genoa, where he remained until his move to Sicily. We know little about Van Dyck's movements between his return to Genoa from Palermo in 1625 and his final return to Antwerp in the autumn of 1627; by early 1628 he had returned to Flanders, never to travel to Italy again. While in Italy Van Dyck produced an astonishing series of paintings, of historical and religious subjects, but his fame mainly rested on portraiture. For a young artist the patronage of personalities such as Cardinal Guido Bentivoglio (fig. 3) would have been particularly important.[5] A full-length portrait of a prince of the Church would have represented an exceptionally prestigious commission for a young foreign painter in Italy. Bentivoglio had been *nunzio* to Flanders and Bellori recorded that when in Rome Van Dyck had stayed with him in his palace on the Quirinal. The portrait of Bentivoglio of circa 1622–23 – one of Van Dyck's absolute achievements in the field of portraiture – is a piece of theatrical display on the painter's part. While the cardinal is suddenly distracted and abandons the reading of a letter, he gazes meditatively into the distance. All the trappings of a state papal portrait, in the tradition of Raphael and Titian, are there: the classical architectural background, the red velvet curtain, a still life of flowers on the table. Bentivoglio's portrait, however, is the ultimate example of sophistication. The cardinal's gown and *mozzetta* of scarlet moiré silk, and the white lace are depicted with astounding technical virtuosity, and the portrait is a masterpiece in terms of painterly effects. The intelligent, melancholic and sensitive air of Bentivoglio, combined with the magnificent demeanour of the figure in the painting, makes this into an archetypal Van Dyck portrait. The seventeenth-century anonymous French compiler of another biography of Van Dyck, based heavily on the letters between Cornelis de Wael in Genoa and Lucas van Uffel in Venice, concluded that after the portrait of Bentivoglio, Van Dyck 'never painted anything that surpassed it. The whole of Rome hastened to see this marvel of art, and everyone wanted to be portrayed by the hand of our artist.'[6]

It is hardly surprising that the Genoese aristocracy flooded the young painter with commissions for grand, full-length portraits. Ladies, in particular, were immortalised by Van Dyck's brush in Genoa – among many examples, the portrait of Elena Grimaldi Cattaneo, painted a year after Cardinal Bentivoglio (fig. 4).[7] The marchesa is outdoors, possibly in the gardens of one of the many villas surrounding Genoa, at Sanpierdarena or Albaro. The architectural background is more sophisticated than the one in Bentivoglio's portrait, with the fluted columns directly quoting sixteenth-century Venetian examples, Paolo Veronese in particular. The black pageboy seems to have stepped out of one of Veronese's *Feasts* as well, but in this case he holds the red parasol to protect Elena's pale complexion.

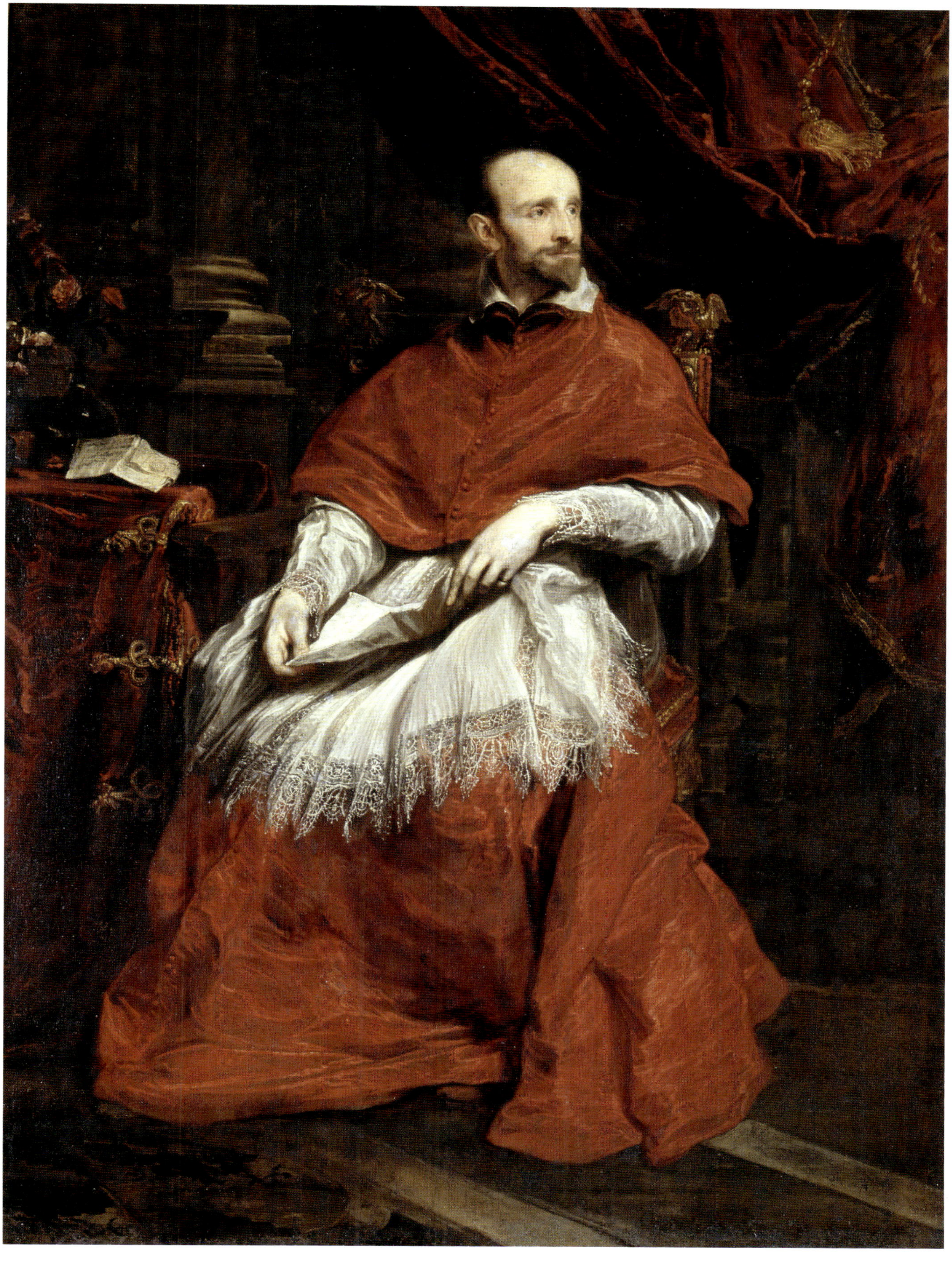

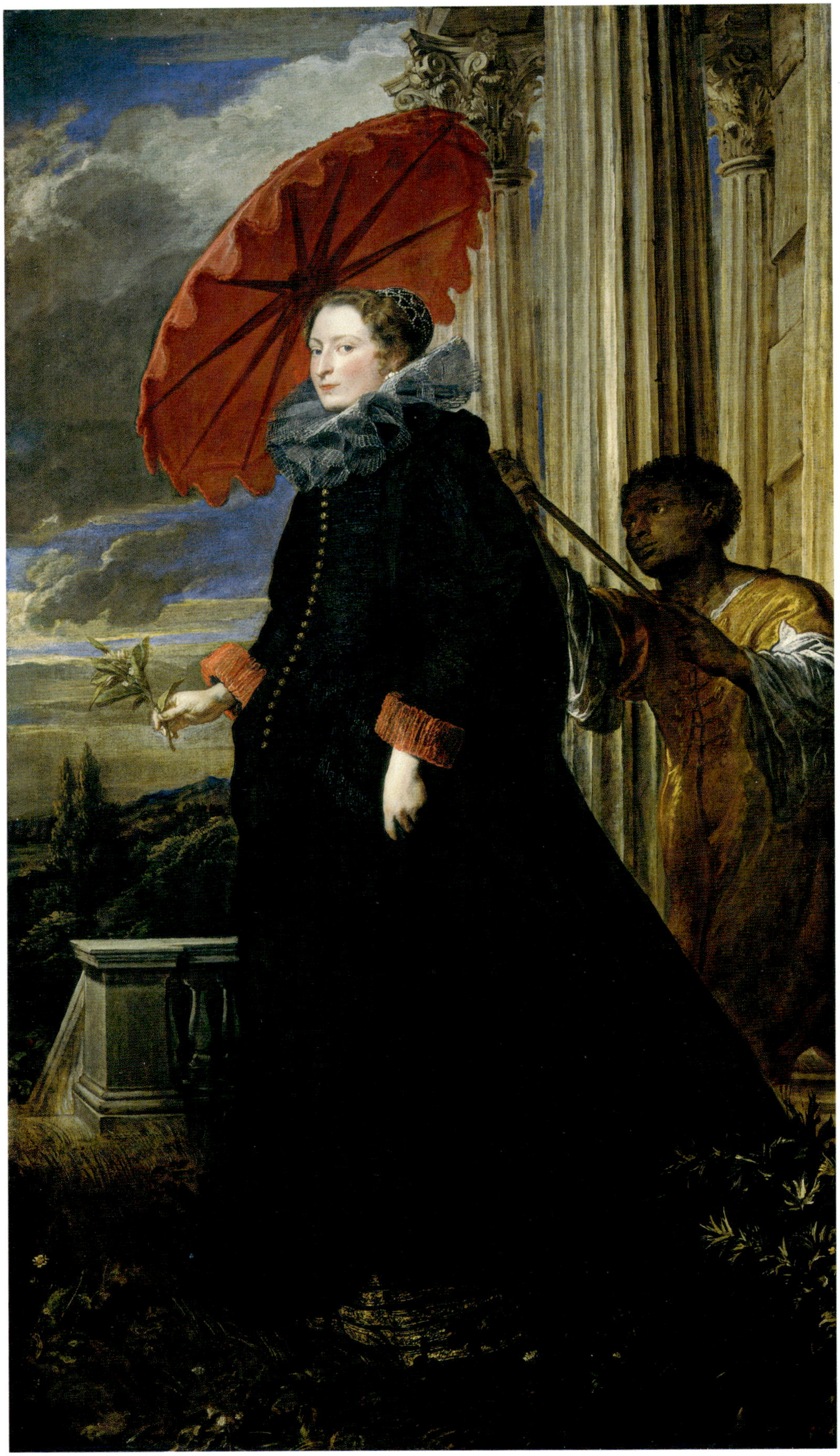

4 | Sir Anthony van Dyck,
Elena Grimaldi Cattaneo
The Widener Collection, Image courtesy of the National Gallery of Art, Washington

5 | Sir Anthony van Dyck,
Portrait of a Boy
Private Collection

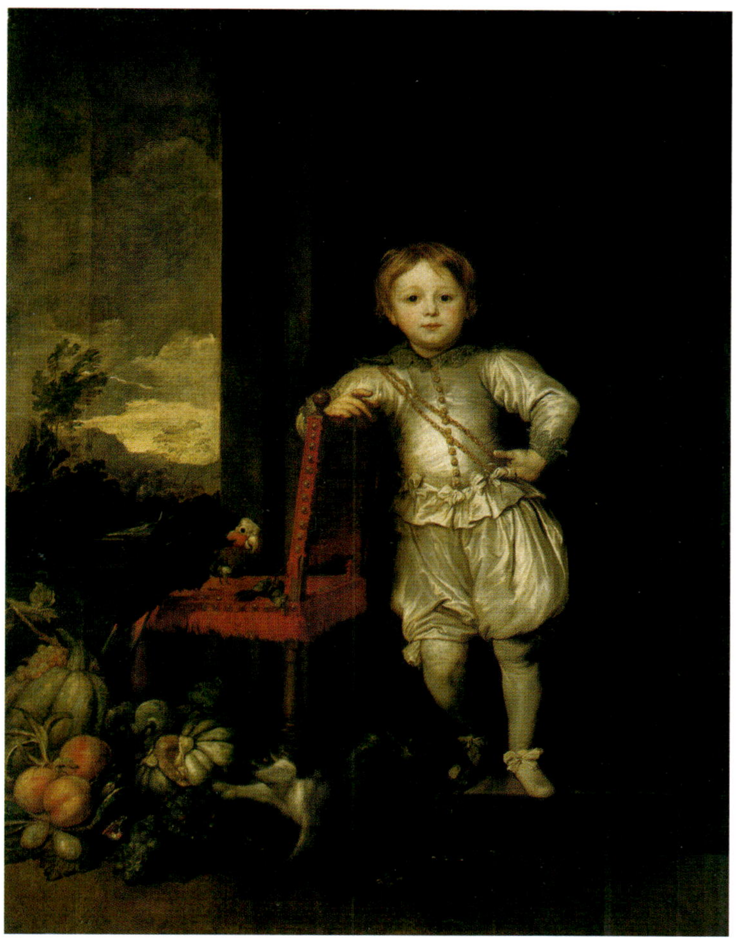

The conceit of the parasol is compositionally successful in drawing the attention to the sitter's handsome face and echoes the red ruffs at the end of the sleeves of her black dress. Elegantly attired, Elena Grimaldi is in this painting the emblematic Genoese noblewoman, with her rich dress and stately appearance. Most extraordinary and still very much in the vein of Titian's example are Van Dyck's portraits of Genoese children. The unidentified boy (fig. 5), in the Durazzo Pallavicini Palace in Genoa, demonstrates how receptive the painter was when portraying very young sitters.[8] The child has the boyish vulnerability of his age but the grand mode of representation suggests an impressive future for the sitter, at the head of a prominent family. The stage setting used for Cardinal Bentivoglio and Elena Grimaldi is used yet again, with the classical architecture and distant landscape, but the overall effect is less formal. In this specific portrait the remarkable still life at the bottom left, with ripe melons, peaches, figs and grapes, the playful monkey stealing fruit, and the parrot on the chair, whose eyes seem to mimic the large, dark eyes of the boy, were the result of Van Dyck's collaboration with the painter Jan Roos. Considering the success of these portraits, especially in Genoa, it is not surprising that the early sources tell us that Van Dyck's move to Sicily was caused by the commission for a portrait.

Sicilian Journey: 1624–25

The main reason for Van Dyck's trip to Palermo seems to have been the prestigious commission for a portrait of the Viceroy of Sicily, Emanuele Filiberto of Savoy (cat. 2). Bellori, in his biography, recorded that 'Anthony conceived a desire to move to Sicily where, as Prince Emanuele Filiberto of Savoy was viceroy at the time, he painted his portrait'.[9] According to the anonymous French biographer, it was Emanuele Filiberto who had invited the painter to Palermo.[10] Van Dyck was probably in Turin, between December 1622 and February 1623, on his way between Venice and Rome, and it is possible that links with the Savoy family were established at such an early date, perhaps through the agency of the Countess of Arundel.[11]

Van Dyck arrived in Palermo in the spring of 1624.[12] The city he reached would have been significantly different from anything

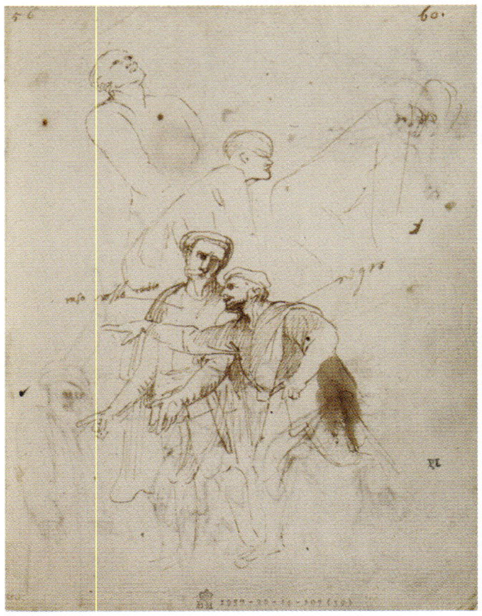

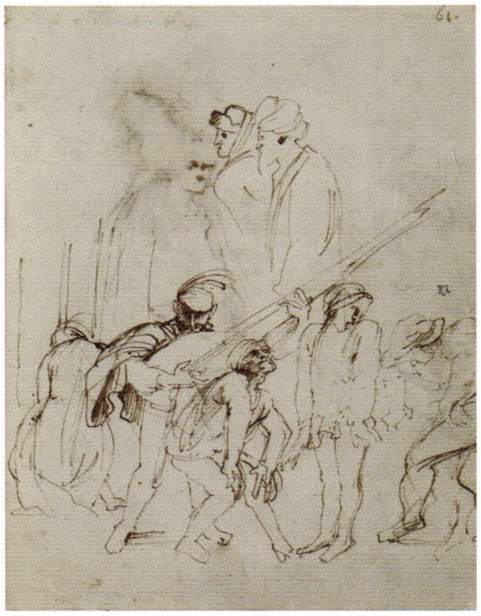

6 | Sir Anthony van Dyck, *Italian Sketchbook – Commedia dell'Arte Performance and Acrobats* The British Museum, London, fol. 59r

7 | Sir Anthony van Dyck, *Italian Sketchbook – Commedia dell'Arte Performance and Lutenist* The British Museum, London, fol. 60r

he had seen before. Palermo was not as large as other cities Van Dyck had visited – the population was about 130,000 people – and not as wealthy as Genoa, but it was geographically, historically and culturally exceptional.[13] The urban fabric spread from the sea and the harbour towards the Cathedral and the Royal Palace. Along the main route were the palaces of the aristocracy and churches, surrounded by the countryside of the Conca d'Oro. The perfume of orange blossoms from the gardens would have welcomed the young Flemish artist to Palermo, a city that still had significant remains from the many civilisations that had colonised it, Greeks, Arabs and Normans in particular. It is not recorded how Van Dyck responded to the golden mosaics and the remnants of mosques, but surely he must have been particularly intrigued by the exotic surroundings provided by Sicily. Seventeenth-century Palermo was also rich in artistic patronage and collecting, and the court around the viceroy was especially attuned to the visual arts.[14]

While in Palermo, Van Dyck was drawn to scenes he witnessed in the streets around him. Very few drawings from the *Italian Sketchbook* (cat. 5) represent contemporary events; of these, a group of three pages depicts acrobats, musicians and actors performing *commedia dell'arte* plays (figs. 6–7).[15] They are likely to have been sketched in Palermo, as in the sketchbook they directly follow a particularly fascinating drawing, inscribed 'a witch in Palermo' (fig. 8).[16] A single, sad figure occupies the left side of the sheet, below the inscription; she is an old, toothless woman dressed in simple robes, with a rope tied with a knot around her neck. She holds a long lit taper, and wears a tall conical hat with a devil drawn onto it. Two other figures are sketched faintly on each side of her. Witchcraft was fiercely fought in seventeenth-century Europe and trials against women accused of it were common. In Sicily the Spanish Inquisition acted with particular force against all types of heresy, and was altogether separate from the Roman Inquisition that had jurisdiction over the rest of Italy.[17] From Inquisition documents we know that Van Dyck could have witnessed in Palermo only one *Auto da Fé* – a mass accompanied by the public punishment of heretics – on 19 May 1624, in the square in front of the church of San Domenico.[18] On such occasions, depending if the heretics repented and were reconciled with the Church or remained obstinate, they were castigated more or less severely. Six people stood in front of the Inquisition that day in Palermo: four bigamists, one blasphemer, and a witch; their names are not recorded, but all six repented. Van Dyck sketched the witch after her trial, the fact that she carries a lit candle identifying her as a repentant heretic. Her punishment is likely to have been flagellation, as only obstinate heretics were condemned to death, and while the artist was in Palermo no such sentences took place. Apart from *commedia dell'arte* figures, musicians and a witch, no other people or sights in the streets of the city were recorded by Van Dyck in his sketchbook.

Palermo hosted an important Flemish community, and his compatriots welcomed Van Dyck in Sicily. Hendrik Dych (or Van Dich), from Antwerp, was the Consul of Flanders and Germany in Palermo, from at least June 1619, and the surname suggests that he may have had family ties with the painter. He was a merchant, stockbroker, importer and collector of art. Together with his business partner, Andrea Rademacher, the consul was involved in the commerce of salt, grain, sulphur and works of art, including tapestries.[19] Dych was linked to people Van Dyck knew well, such as the Van Uffel brothers and Genoese families, like the Pilo and Della Torre. Sicilians, furthermore, had a particular taste in the seventeenth century for Flemish art. A few Northern artists are, in fact, documented in Palermo when Van Dyck visited the city.[20] Willem Walsgart arrived in Sicily in 1612; Gaspar de Momper was in Palermo in 1619, even though he was not likely there for a long time; and Jan Basquens and Hieronymus Gerards were in the city from the early 1620s. Jan Brueghel the Younger also visited Palermo between 1623 and the summer of 1625.[21]

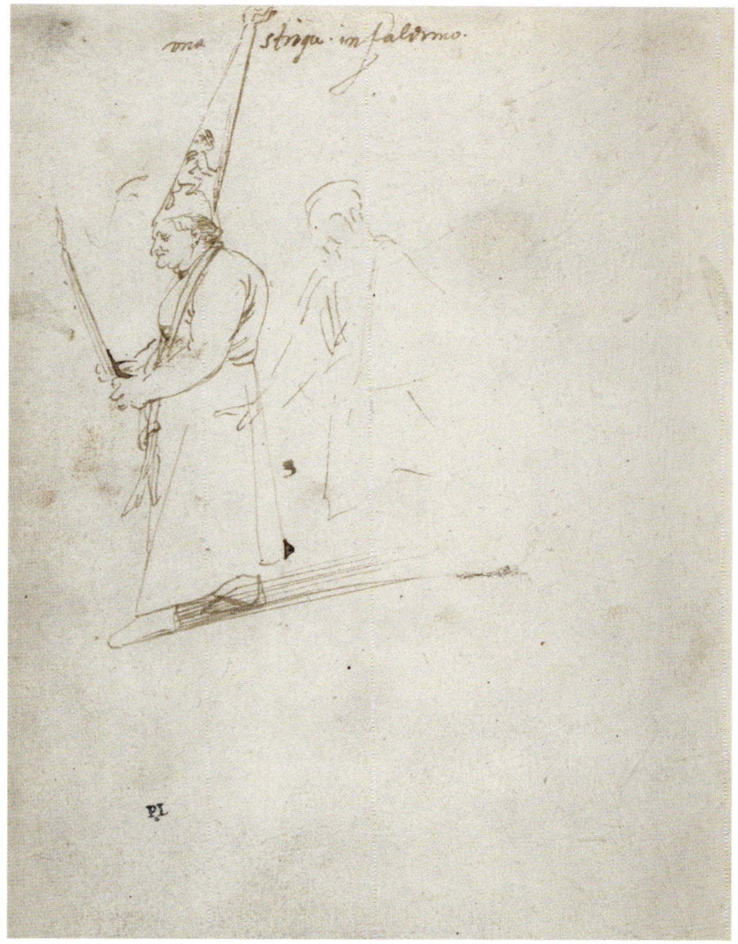

8 | Sir Anthony van Dyck,
Italian Sketchbook – A Witch in Palermo
The British Museum, London, fol. 58v

When travelling in Italy, Van Dyck usually stayed with friends and people he knew – the De Wael brothers in Genoa, Cardinal Bentivoglio in Rome – and in Palermo he followed a similar example and was Hendrik Dych's guest. The consul's house, now destroyed, was next to the church of Santa Maria di Portosalvo (fig. 9) on the Strada del Cassaro, between the harbour and the main road that connected the seafront with the Cathedral. Van Dyck paid 80 *onze* per year as a lodger in the large house; according to the documents the building had a view over the Cala and the city harbour ('*cum prospettiva ex parte maris*').[22] It is not known, however, where the artist worked, and if he had a studio set up in Palermo; it is likely that Dych's house also functioned as a working space for Van Dyck.

The Flemish community was not the only foreign group of people in Palermo that the painter was connected with. The city was also home to a large number of Genoese merchants, and many of them would have provided the logical social bridge for Van Dyck between Genoa and Palermo.[23] The Genoese were grouped around their national church, San Giorgio dei Genovesi (fig. 10), which had been decorated at the beginning of the seventeenth century with paintings by Filippo Paladini, Bernardo Castello and Palma il Giovane.[24] Two of Van Dyck's patrons in Palermo were prominent members of the Genoese community, closely involved with the church of San Giorgio, and both owned chapels there: Desiderio Segno (cat. 8) and Orazio Lomellini, the husband of Sofonisba Anguissola (cats. 5–7). Segno was consul of the Genoese community from at least November 1623 to December 1624, and Lomellini subsequently from April 1625 to May 1626.[25]

In recent years a significant group of documents has been discovered, shedding new light on Van Dyck's stay in Palermo. They reveal a close network of people between the Flemish and Genoese communities that the artist was closely involved with. The first mention of the painter in the city comes from his own sketchbook (cat. 5), where his visit to the old painter Sofonisba Anguissola is dated 12 July 1624, only a few months after his arrival in Sicily. On 21 November of that year, Van Dyck appeared as 'Flemish painter, at present living in Palermo' ('*Antonius van dych quoq[ue] pittor fiamenghus et ad p[raese]ns hic pan[ormi] degens*'), and acted as guarantor for Jan Brueghel the Younger having received 19 *onze* from Hendrik Dych on the previous 29 July.[26] Two other witnesses to the transaction were the Genoese Clemente Pilo and the Flemish Hector Vanachtoven. According to Francesco Susinno, Van Dyck knew Vanachtoven well and stayed with him in Messina, probably that summer. In his life of the Flemish artist Jan van Houbraken, published in 1724, Susinno recorded that Vanachtoven, who was at that time considered one of the richest merchants in Messina and a man of impeccable taste ('*in quel tempo stimato il più ricco mercante ed uomo di gusto molto delicato*'), called Van Dyck from Palermo especially ('*fe' venire apposta da Palermo Antonio van Eix [sic]*') to commission two portraits, half-figures, one of himself and the other of his wife ('*per farsi fare dui ritratti, uno per sé e l'altro per sua moglie, in mezze figure*').[27] Susinno recorded that Vanachtoven's son-in-law, the Marchese di Penticattilo, left these two portraits to the Marqués del Carpio, when he was transferred from Ambassador in Rome to Viceroy of Naples.[28] Except from Susinno's mention, however, Van Dyck's possible stay in Messina and the portraits

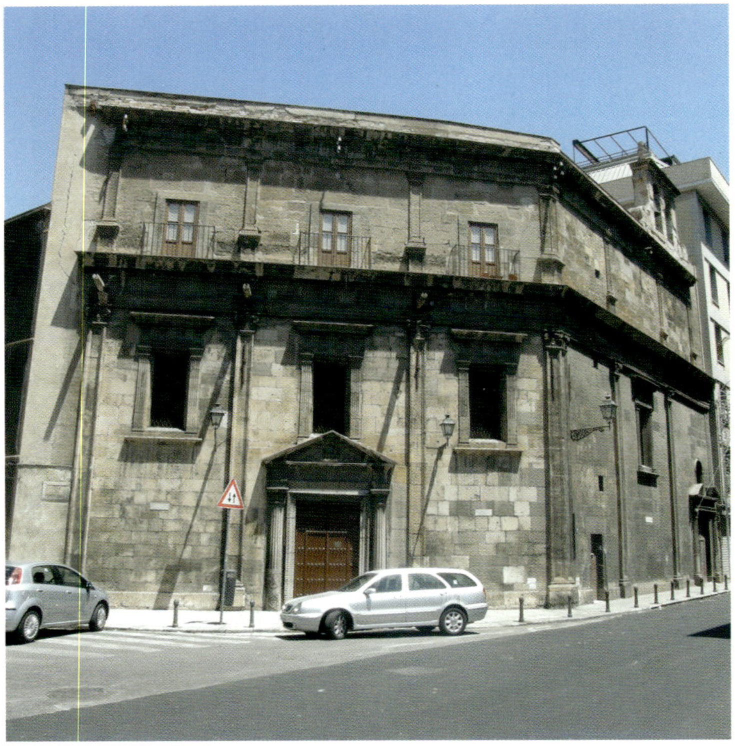

9 | Santa Maria di Portosalvo, Palermo

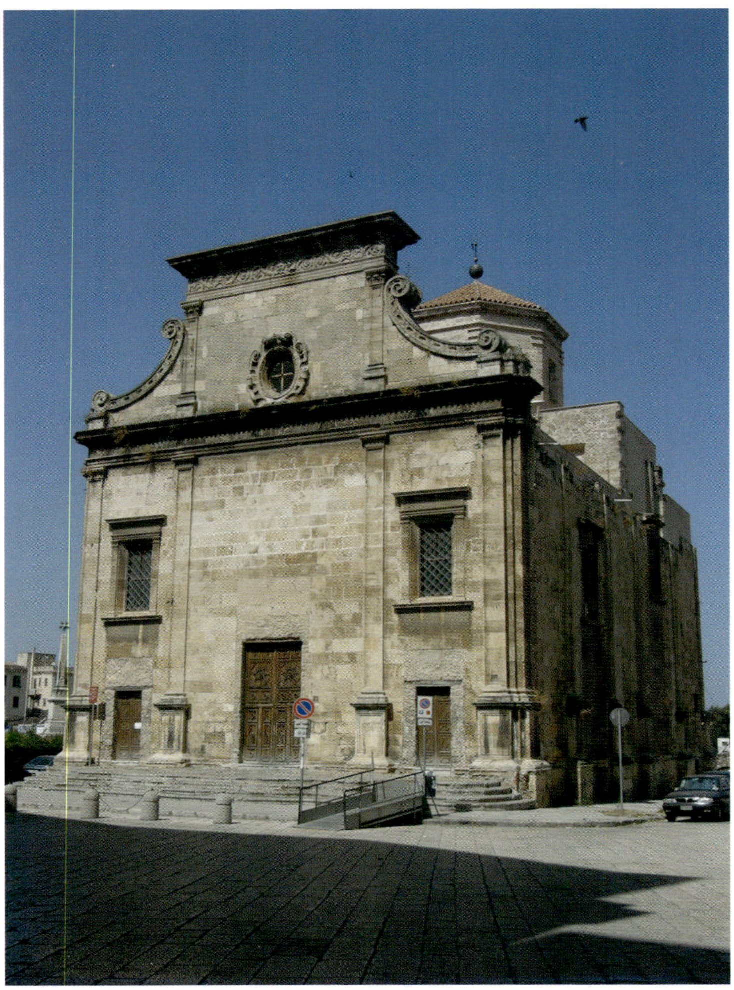

10 | San Giorgio dei Genovesi, Palermo

of Vanachtoven and his wife are not otherwise documented.

More documents add to our knowledge of Van Dyck's relations with the Flemish Consul Dych. On 6 April 1625, Van Dyck declared to have received 36 *onze* and 12 *tari* from Dych; the bill of exchange was sent to Cornelis de Wael in Genoa.[29] A note to the document adds that as the bill of exchange was not accepted, Hector Vanachtoven, on behalf of Dych, received the money directly from Van Dyck on 20 August of that year. Another document, also of 6 April 1625, reveals that the painter was also producing works in Palermo in exchange for hospitality. Van Dyck and Dych declared themselves satisfied 'for all the food he [Dych] had given him [Van Dyck] at his home, the said Van Dyck promised the same Dych all the paintings he had hitherto made for him' ('*de o[mn]ibus alimentis per eum sibi prestitis in eius domo et d[ittus] de vandych ab eodem de dich stip[ulan]te de o[mn]ibus picturis per eum factis d[ict]o de dich usque ad p[raese]ns*').[30] It has been suggested that one of these paintings may have been a portrait of Dych himself.[31] Two of the paintings Van Dyck made for Dych were *Crucifixions*, as recorded in another document of 7 May 1625. Van Dyck declared to have received 4 *onze* from Clemente Pilo who had promised to pay the said four *onze* 'for the execution by the said Van Dyck of a painting of the Crucifixion for Hendrik Dych, who is now in the possession of the said painting' ('*per manifattura d'un quatro con figura dello Crocifisso per d[itt]o di vandich fatto ad Henrico Dych quale hoggi e in potere dello d[itt]o di Dych*').[32] Another 6 *onze* were added 'for a painting with the image of the crucified Christ made for him [Dych] by himself [Van Dyck] and delivered at an earlier date' ('*pro manifactura unius quatri cum Immagine Crucifissi per eum sibi facti et consig[na]ti t[emp]oribus pret[eritis]*'). While in Palermo, Van Dyck was still being paid for Genoese commissions: on 18 August 1625 the painter declared to have received 10 *onze* from Jacopo and Giovanni Battista Brignone, through a bill of exchange from Giovanni Battista Cattaneo that was issued in Genoa on 23 May.[33] The money was

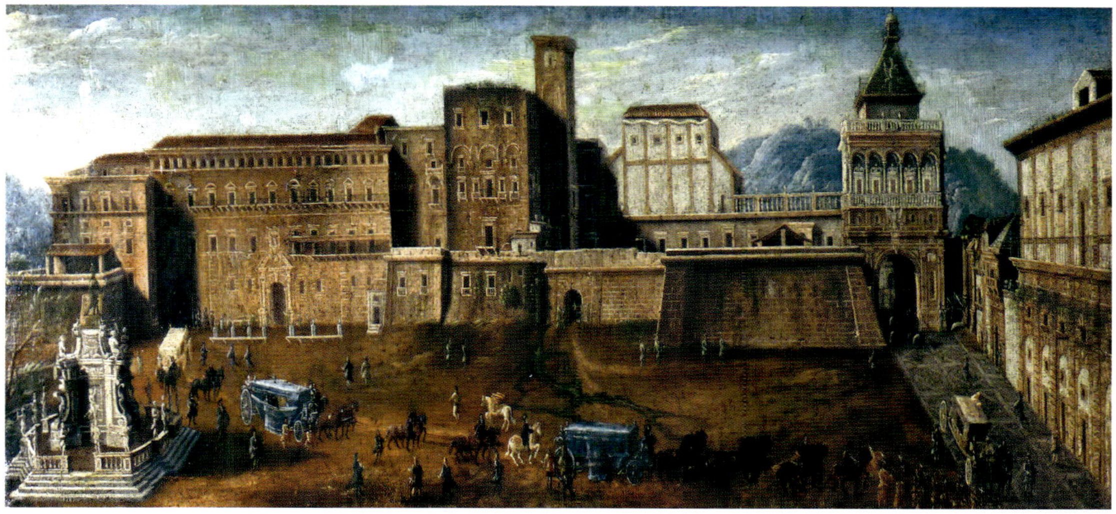

11 | Anonymous, *Royal Palace (Palazzo dei Normanni) in Palermo*
Museo Pepoli, Trapani

possibly for one or more of the family portraits that Van Dyck had painted for the Cattaneo family.

A further document of 3 September 1625, shortly before Van Dyck left Sicily, records more of his works made in Sicily and now lost.[34] The artist granted Hieronymus Gerards the power of attorney to repossess various paintings from Domenico Martinetto, who had been Van Dyck's servant ('*creato*') in Palermo. The pictures listed, presumably by Van Dyck, were sketches in oil on paper of 'a head of a young man named Baldassaro with black curly hair, a head of Simon disguised as a woman, a head of a sailor, a head of Saint Peter, a head of a woman with loose hair, a head of Lucia with a firm breast, a satirical head of a reader and a head shouting with mouth open' ('*una testa d'un Gioven nominato Baldassaro con li capelli nigri et rizzi una testa di simuni fatta à guisa di donna una testa di marinaro una testa di san Petro una testa d'una donna con li capilli sparsi una testa di lucia co lu pettu rigido una testa di lettore alla satiresca et una testa che grida con la bocca aperta*'). This is the only evidence of Van Dyck's workshop practice in Palermo, and what the young Martinetto (servant or apprentice) must have stolen were sketches produced by the painter in the studio to use for larger historical or religious compositions.

The Viceroy: Emanuele Filiberto of Savoy

When Van Dyck arrived in Sicily, the viceroy – most probably the man who had invited him to Palermo – was Emanuele Filiberto of Savoy. Eleven years older than the Flemish painter, the viceroy was born in Turin in 1588, and had moved to Sicily only two years before Van Dyck, in February 1622.[35] He was the third son of Duke Carlo Emanuele I of Savoy who, in 1585, had married the Infanta Catalina Micaela, daughter of King Philip II of Spain. Most of Emanuele Filiberto's life was spent in the service of the Spanish crown. After a first trip to Spain between 1603 and 1606, with his brothers Filippo Emanuele and Vittorio Amedeo, he moved there permanently in 1610. From 1600 he was Grand Prior of Castille for the Knights of Malta and the king made him admiral of the Spanish fleet (*Capitán General del Mar*) in 1612. His father gave him the title of Prince of Oneglia in 1620. In 1622, King Philip IV nominated him Viceroy of Sicily and upon landing there, Emanuele Filiberto embarked on public projects for the island. Most importantly he created a series of buildings – the so-called Palazzata – along the waterfront of the harbour of Messina.

In Palermo, the viceroy's interests converged in the area around his residence, the Royal Palace (or Palazzo dei Normanni – fig. 11). The Ospedale di San Giacomo was built between the palace and the Cathedral, and parts of the palace itself were re-worked.[36] A gallery was instituted above the palace's Porta Nuova, an armoury was established, and a room was created for the newly founded Accademia dei Riaccesi. The mathematician Carlo Maria Ventimiglia, one of the key Sicilian intellectuals of the day, headed the Accademia as '*principe*'. Emanuele Filiberto was above all interested in the arts, as demonstrated by the inventories of his possessions compiled after his death.[37] In his Gallery at the Palazzo dei Normanni, the viceroy assembled a series of portraits of the Savoy and Spanish royal families, including images of kings of Spain (Charles V, Philip II, Philip III and Philip IV) and a series of thirty-eight large oval pictures of hermits.[38] These types of paintings clearly demonstrated a particularly Spanish influence, and were directly related to similar canvases in the palace of the Buen Retiro in Madrid and in the convent of the Descalzas Reales. The picture gallery of the Royal Palace in Palermo included more than two hundred paintings. They were mostly portraits and religious scenes. Only few of the viceroy's paintings have been identified – among them Francesco Bassano's *Adam in the Earthly Paradise* (fig. 12). Emanuele Filiberto was seen as an important patron by contemporary artists; in 1624, from Naples, Jusepe de Ribera dedicated to the viceroy an etching of the

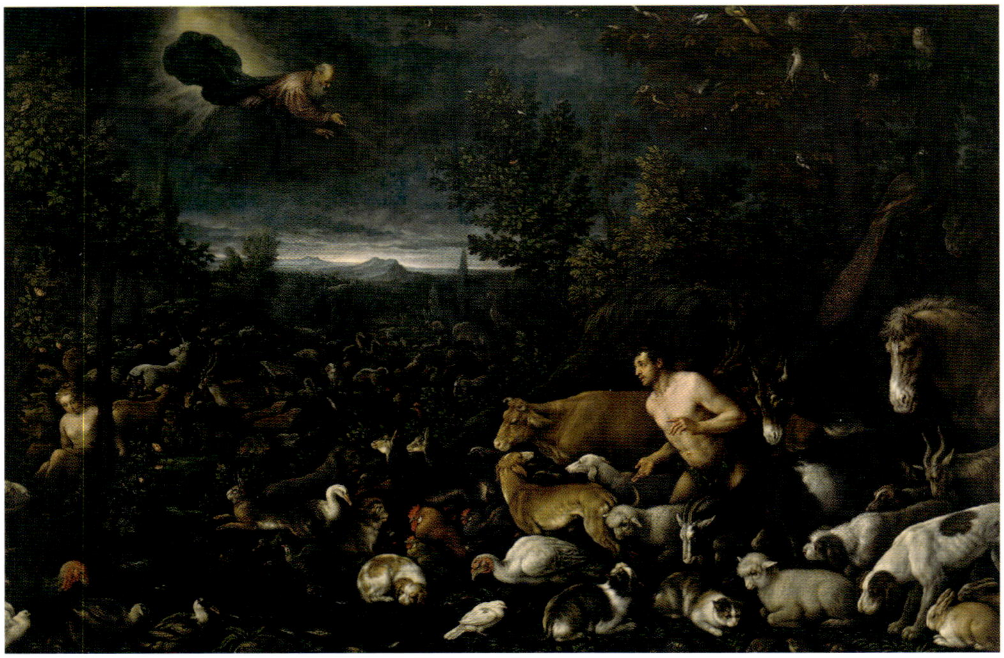

12 | Francesco Bassano,
Adam in the Earthly Paradise
Museo Nacional del Prado, Madrid

Martyrdom of Saint Bartholomew (fig. 13), most likely trying to establish a foundation for future patronage. Van Dyck's portrait of Emanuele Filiberto (cat. 2) was probably commissioned for the Royal Palace, but it is unrecorded before 1793. The painting is likely to be the portrait that Giovan Francesco Fiocchetto, the viceroy's personal doctor, wrote about in his 1628 biography of Emanuele Filiberto. According to Fiocchetto, the viceroy had sat for a portrait, which was then placed on one of the walls of the Guardaroba ('*cubiculo mosaico*') in the so-called Sala del Mosaico of the palace (fig. 14).[39] Emanuele Filiberto used to spend time alone in that room and no one except for him was allowed in the Sala. One day, returning from mass, the viceroy entered the room and found his portrait face down on the floor. As this could have not been caused by any natural occurrence, he took it as an ill omen.

The palace's gallery also included a significant collection of books and scientific instruments. Globes and clocks demonstrated Emanuele Filiberto's scientific interests, and in its installation the collection probably followed the examples of Philip II's Library at El Escorial and the Grande Galleria of Carlo Emanuele I in Turin.[40] Carlo Maria Ventimiglia, in his funeral eulogy, wrote that the viceroy 'was also most knowledgeable in moral, political and natural sciences, and furthermore Filiberto became excellent in mathematics, a science in which most good men are idle, and just one person in every century is successful in it, whereas in other sciences innumerable men are expert; and even in mechanics, and he operated in that with his own hands [...] the nautical charts, and the other infinite instruments by him envisaged and made, bear witness also to him and more than any other fallen ornament they celebrate his glory'.[41] The armoury of the Royal Palace in Palermo seems to have also been particularly rich.[42] It was housed on the first floor of the palace, above the Cavallerizza and towards the Porta Nuova. It was modelled on Philip II's Real Armería in Madrid and included, among many pieces, the armour designed by the Maestro dal Castello for the viceroy (cat. 3). Emanuele Filiberto's collection, as demonstrated by the inventories, also included precious objects – diamonds were particularly fashionable in Spain and Sicily at the time – and textiles.[43]

Pestilence and Death

A few months after Van Dyck reached Palermo and as soon as the viceroy's portrait was finished, the plague hit the city. The first symptoms of the pestilence were recorded on 7 May 1624 and the epidemic continued until June 1626. The account of Capitano Maya of what happened in the city is particularly detailed.[44] The beginning of the plague in the city was blamed on a ship that had arrived from Tunis in May; with it, it was said, the pestilence had entered the harbour of Palermo.[45] By 15 June many people were dying throughout Palermo and soon casualties were also found in the Royal Palace.[46] A crucifix was brought in procession from the Cathedral to the church of Santa Maria della Catena, near the harbour, for two consecutive days, but with no significant results; by June the doors to the city were closed and no one could leave or enter Palermo.[47] Emanuele Filiberto issued an official letter on 25 June to announce the state of emergency, and a network was immediately set up to control the plague, with *deputati* in charge of the situation, and *lazzaretti* where the sick and dead were collected.[48] It was calculated that between May and December 1624 more than ten thousand people died in Palermo alone.[49] The committee of the Deputazione della Sanità was created to oversee the situation and block the spread of the plague in any possible way. A *bando*

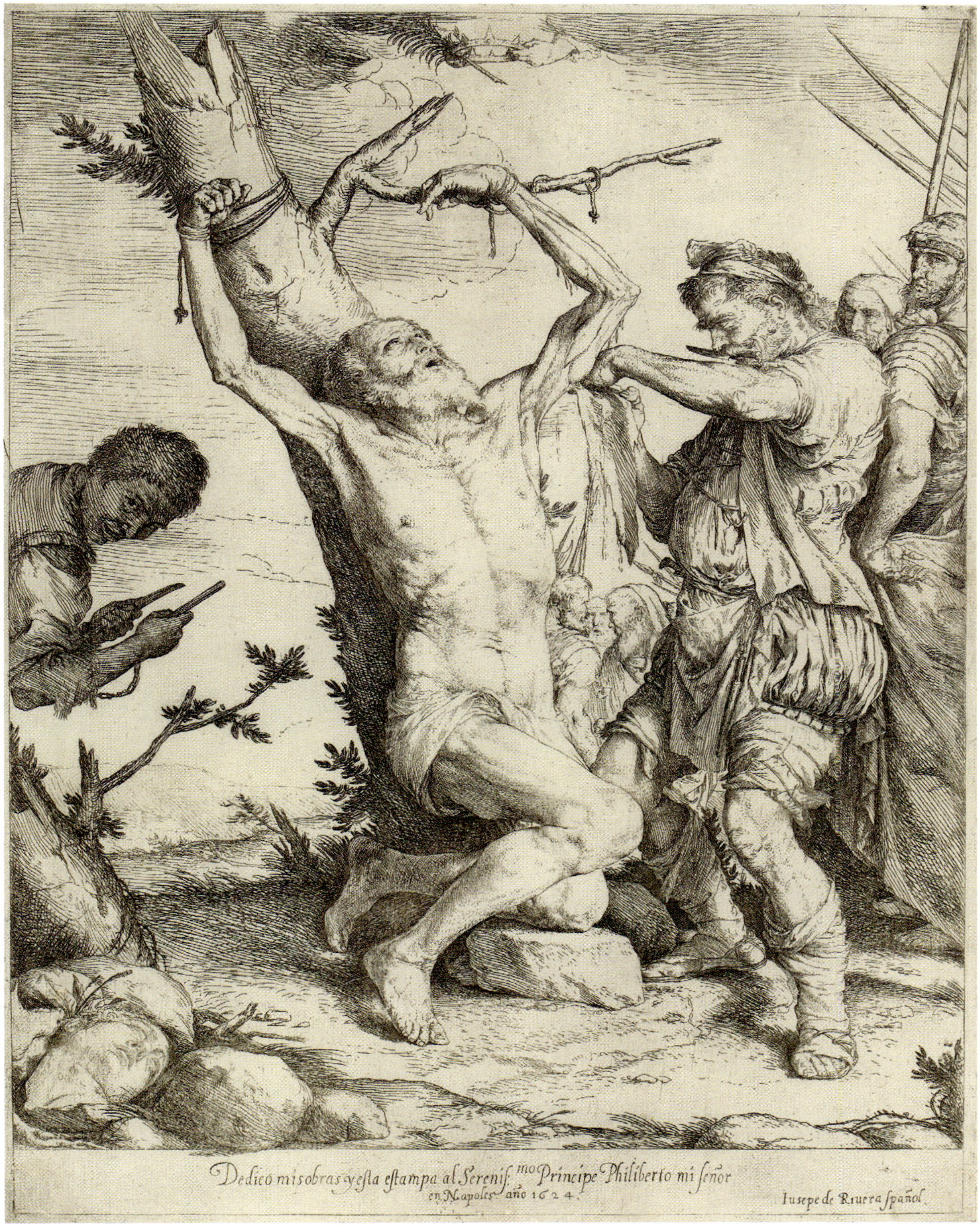
Dedico mis obras y esta estampa al Serenis.mo Principe Philiberto mi señor
en Napoles año 1624.
Iusepe de Riuera spañol

13 | Jusepe de Ribera,
Martyrdom of Saint Bartholomew
The British Museum, London

of 1625 issued by the Deputazione outlined the general rules to combat the pestilence.[50] No one was allowed into the city of Palermo, no matter where they came from, unless they had with them an official document ('*bollettino*') proving their health.[51] If visitors were found at the city doors and harbour without the '*bollettino*' they were not allowed entrance; if an illegal visitor was found in Palermo he was to be condemned to fustigation and a period of seven years in the royal galleys, if a woman the galleys were to be commuted for four months' working at the hospital of La Cuba, the main *lazzaretto* of the city.[52] If the unlawful tourist was a nobleman he was to pay a fine of 100 *onze* and to be imprisoned for seven years in a castle to be determined.[53] As soon as someone was found ill anywhere in the city, it had to be declared to one of the *deputati* within twenty-four hours, and they had to be sent to the hospital of La Cuba, unless too ill to leave the house.

Notwithstanding all possible precautions, the city was soon in total chaos and it was obvious that the plague was out of control. On 28 July 1624, the viceroy himself left the palace to inspect the city; he travelled in his carriage from the Royal Palace to Porta Felice. By the time he had returned to the palace, he was ill.[54] A procession brought the relics of Saint Christina from the Cathedral to the bed of the sick

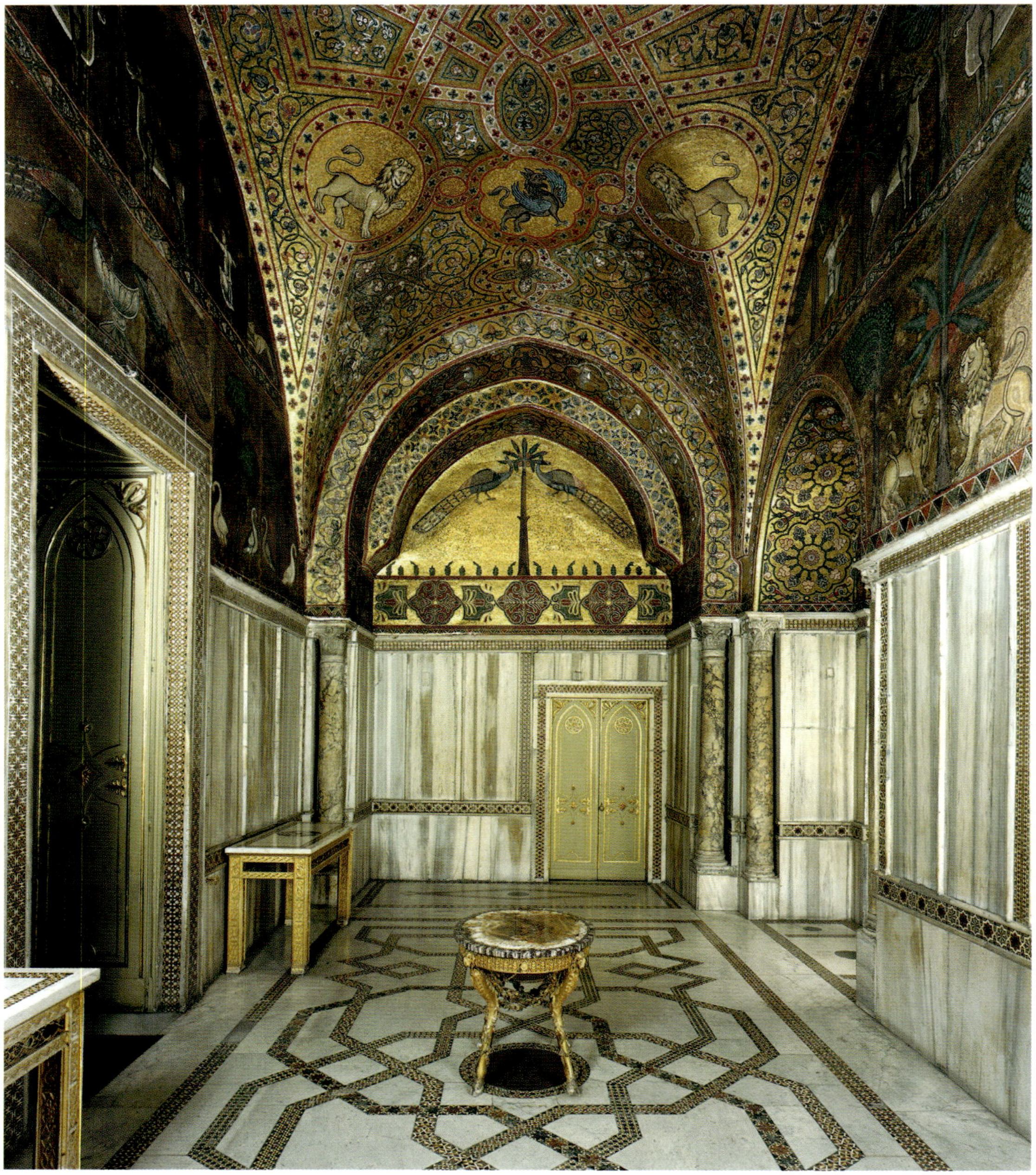

14 | Sala del Mosaico, Royal Palace, Palermo

viceroy, together with a painting of Saint Rosalia that belonged to the Jesuits.[55] On 3 August, despite the cures of Giovan Francesco Fiocchetto, the physician whom the viceroy had brought with him from Turin, Emanuele Filiberto died in the Royal Palace. At the end of the month, on 26 and 27 August, a solemn funeral was held in the Cathedral for the viceroy (fig. 15), with especially designed decorations, and a eulogy written by Carlo Maria Ventimiglia.[56]

The death of Emanuele Filiberto – at that date unmarried and without children – created significant issues in terms of his inheritance. The thirty-six-year-old viceroy had written a will, in which he designated his sister Isabella of Savoy, wife of Alfonso d'Este, Duke of Modena, as universal heiress.[57] Emanuele Filiberto's assets were significant, as it had been agreed with his brothers that all the material possessions of their mother, the Infanta Catilina Micaela, would go uniquely to him. The will was not signed and legally in the case of plague this should not have mattered. However, Carlo Emanuele I, Emanuele Filiberto's father, contested the will, trying to reclaim his son's possessions for Turin, against his own daughter the Duchess of Modena. Fiocchetto, the viceroy's doctor defended the Duke of Savoy's interests and tried to prove that the viceroy had not died of the plague, but simply of *febbre quartana*, rendering the will null and void. With Emanuele Filiberto's death and the plague, Sicily was without a ruler, and the Archbishop of Palermo, the Genoese Giannettino Doria, took control of the political situation. In matters to do with the viceroy's inheritance he was to play a major role. By the autumn of 1624, the Duke and Duchess of Modena had sent ambassadors to

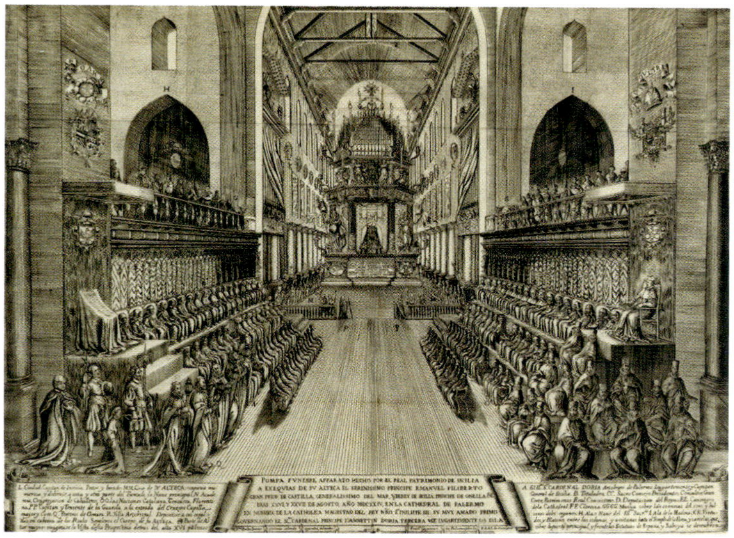

15 | Funeral of Emanuele Filiberto of Savoy from F. Roales, *Exequias del Serenissimo Principe Emanuele Filiberto* Biblioteca Reale, Turin

16 | Tomb of Emanuele Filiberto of Savoy, Panteón de los Infantes, El Escorial

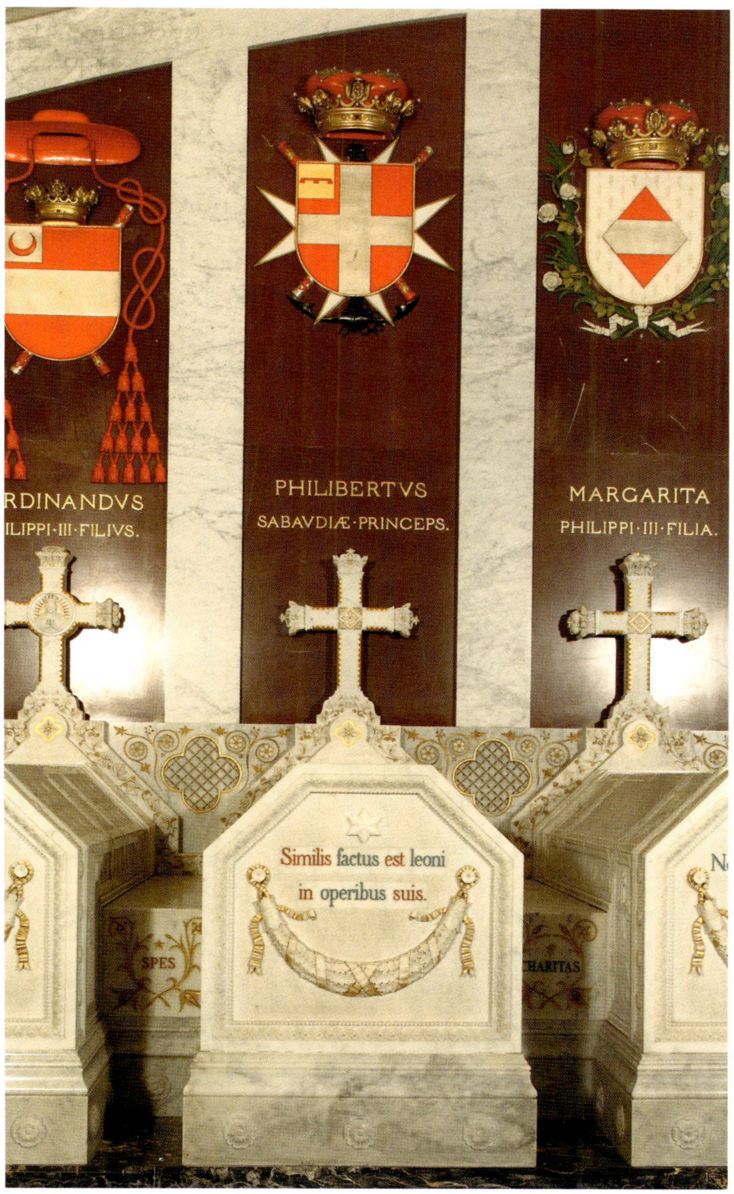

Sicily to reclaim the rightful inheritance. The Modenese ambassador Giovanni Cortesi wrote back from Messina on 4 November that 'all possessions are still in the palace, untouched, under the careful vigilance of Cardinal Doria, but I cannot say what the situation to do with inventories is, or even who compiled them'.[58] By this point it was impossible to enter Palermo because of the quarantine, but Cortesi declared himself 'most determined to go there, so that Your Highness can be informed of every matter'.[59] In the afternoon of 24 November, Cortesi reached Palermo: 'On the bank where we disembarked a huge number of people had gathered, as it seemed to them a miracle to see what in the situation of these most miserable times rarely can be seen, that is that people are coming into that city from where they would gladly leave to escape its dangers.'[60] Even though they were in the city, the Modenese ambassadors were not allowed into the palace, with the excuse that the plague there was still contagious. Cardinal Doria insisted that the duke and duchess, together with the inheritance, would have to be in charge of the dead viceroy's debts as well, but as it was unclear what the assets were, and the envoys could not inspect Emanuele Filiberto's belongings, they soon decided that it was not worth their efforts.[61] The ambassadors sent back their reports and returned to Modena. An inventory of the viceroy's possessions, probably incomplete, and with no valuations, compiled between 8 August and 11 November 1624 was sent to Modena.[62] The collection of Emanuele Filiberto began to be dispersed over the next summer. The gallery of the palace was emptied and, between 11 June and 9 August 1625, the collection was sold at auction in Palermo, under the auspices of Cardinal Doria.[63] The list of objects sold in 1625 demonstrates that many items had already gone missing since the inventory of 1624. Philip IV of Spain and Carlo Emanuele I of Savoy, together with Giannettino Doria, must have organised this, as many objects eventually reached Madrid and Turin. On 2 September 1625, a ship sailed from Palermo to Spain with the body of Emanuele Filiberto on it; the boat, in fact, was also loaded with some of his most treasured possessions. These

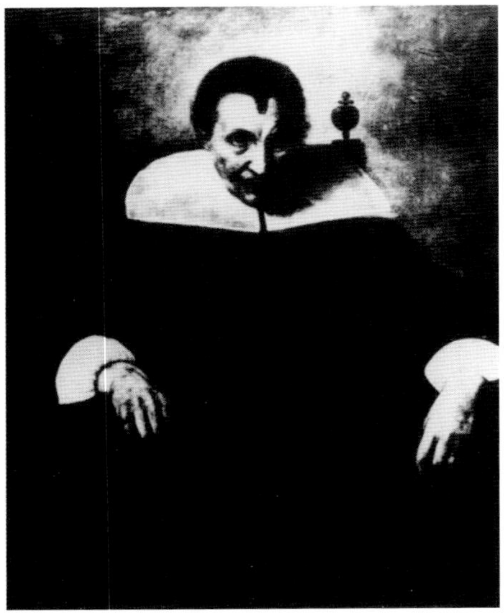

17 | Dutch School,
Portrait of a Woman
Unknown location

18 | Tomb of Sofonisba Anguissola,
San Giorgio dei Genovesi, Palermo

19 | Segno Chapel, San Giorgio
dei Genovesi, Palermo

included some of his paintings (such as the Bassano – fig. 12) and armours (cat. 3).[64] On 22 December 1625, the body of Emanuele Filiberto was buried at El Escorial, in the royal family's burial chambers (fig. 16).[65]

'*Illustres mundi mulieres*': the Painter Sofonisba Anguissola

As the plague was beginning to hit Palermo, and just a few weeks before the viceroy died, Van Dyck paid an important visit to another artist living in the city. On 12 July 1624 he went to see the aged painter Sofonisba Anguissola. Born in Cremona, from an aristocratic family, Sofonisba had trained as a painter and moved to Spain in 1559 as lady-in-waiting to Philip II's new queen, Elizabeth of Valois. Between 1568 and 1572 Sofonisba lived in Madrid, where she had given painting lessons to the Infantas Catalina Micaela (Emanuele Filiberto's mother) and Isabella Clara Eugenia.[66] Sofonisba had married, in 1573, the Sicilian aristocrat Fabrizio Moncada and had moved with him to the island.[67] For six years they were based in Moncada's fief of Paternò, close to Catania. After her husband's death, in 1579, Sofonisba married the Genoese merchant Orazio Lomellini. Together they moved to Genoa, where they lived for thirty-five years, before returning to Sicily in 1615. Their residence in Palermo was a house on the strada del Piliere, next to the church of Santa Maria del Piliere and not far away from San Giorgio dei Genovesi ('*domus magna in contrata di lo Pileri*').[68] With her husband, Sofonisba had become one of the key figures in the Genoese community in Palermo.

Van Dyck's visit to Sofonisba on 12 July was not necessarily his first or last call on the painter, but it was recorded in detail in his sketchbook (cat. 5). A long inscription in Italian, in Van Dyck's own hand, describes the details of the encounter, next to a drawing of her: 'Portrait of the painter Signora Sofonisba, done from life in Palermo in the year 1624, on 12 July: her age being 96 years, still with her memory and brain most quick, and most kind, and although she has lost her sight because of her old age, she enjoyed to have paintings put in front of her, and with great effort by placing her nose close to the picture, she could make out a little of it, and she took great pleasure in that. As I was doing her portrait, she gave me various recommendations, of not to take the light too high, so that the shadows in the wrinkles of old age should not be too strong, and many other good suggestions. And she also told me part of the story of her life, from which I learnt that she was a painter from nature and a miraculous one, and her greatest misfortune was that she could not paint any longer because of her lack of eyesight: even though her hand was still firm and with no tremor whatsoever.'[69] It is a touching account of the encounter between a twenty-five-year-old painter and a colleague of legendary fame. In a few sentences Van Dyck records his impressions of Sofonisba and the useful advice she gave him in terms of painting portraits. It is unclear what the '*quadro*' that Van Dyck put in front of her was; the only documented painting executed by him before July 1624 in Palermo was the portrait of the viceroy, but it is highly unlikely that he would have carried it with him to Sofonisba's house on the strada del Piliere.

The identification of the '*ritratto*' that Van Dyck made of Sofonisba is also uncertain. The most likely option is that this was the drawing in the sketchbook itself, rather than a painting. The small canvas at Knole (cat. 6) derives from this sketch, but it is impossible to determine if this was made from life in front of Sofonisba, or was subsequently reworked in the artist's studio from the drawing. The idea that Van Dyck produced an 'official' portrait of Sofonisba after his visit is usually supported by the link with a painting from the Nauta collection in Amsterdam, now lost and only known from black and white images (fig. 17).[70] Notwithstanding the general similarity between the features of Sofonisba, as she appears in Van Dyck's *Italian Sketchbook* (cat. 5) and in the painting at Knole (cat. 6), and the

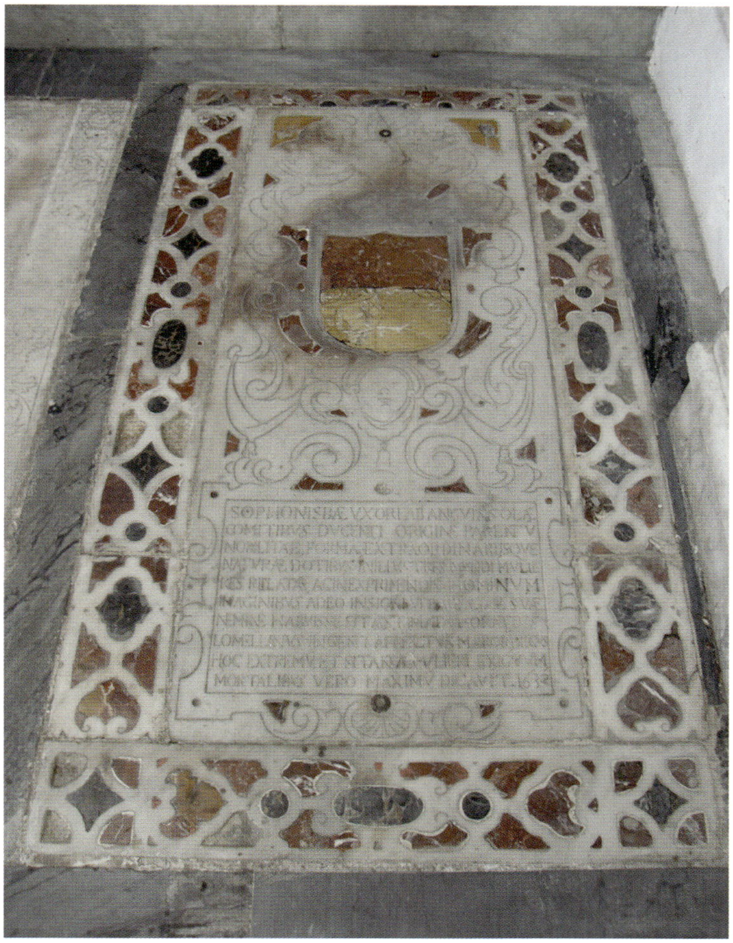

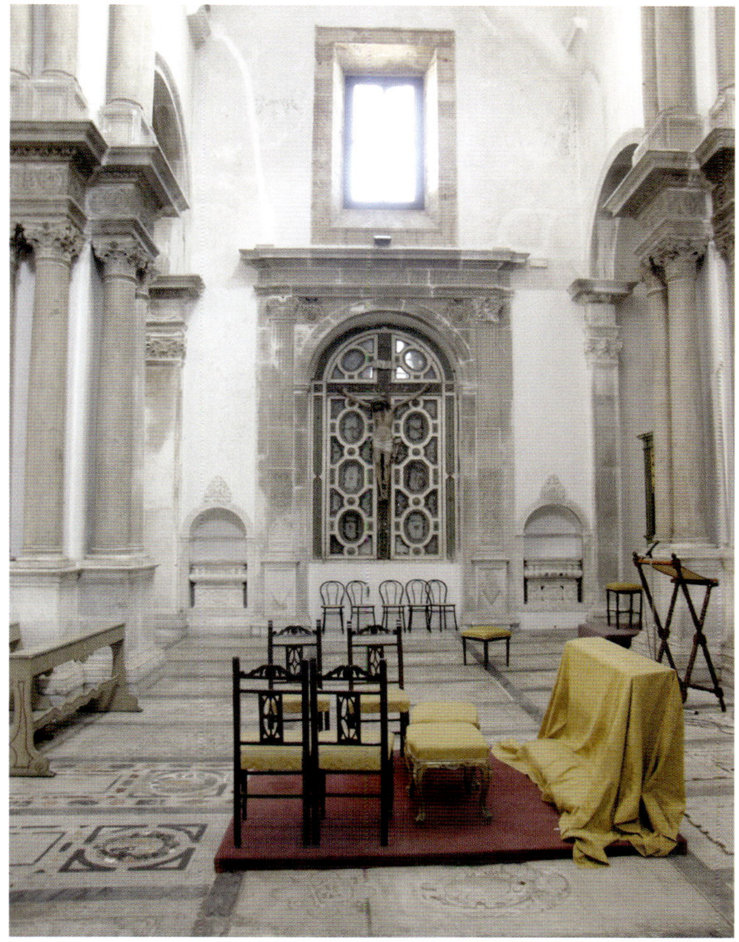

sitter in the ex-Nauta painting, it seems that the latter picture does not represent the female painter. Stylistically the Nauta painting is far from Van Dyck's pictures and is likely to be the work of a Dutch artist that has nothing to do with Van Dyck's Sicilian period.

Sofonisba died on 16 November 1625, soon after Van Dyck left Sicily. It has been suggested that Van Dyck was present at her deathbed and painted Sofonisba one last time.[71] There is no evidence, however, for any contact between the two painters beyond the visit of 12 July 1624, and Van Dyck is last documented in Palermo on 3 September 1625. The painting in Turin, said to represent Sofonisba on her deathbed, even though it has been attributed to Van Dyck in the past, is not by the artist and it is unclear if it represents Sofonisba at all (cat. 7). Sofonisba was buried in San Giorgio dei Genovesi and her husband, years later, had a poignant inscription placed over her tomb (fig. 18): 'Orazio Lomellini, anguished by immense grief, dedicated this extreme honour, indeed most impressive for mortals, but inadequate if dedicated to such a woman, to his wife Sofonisba, descendant of the Counts of Anguissola, considered among the famous women of the century for her noble birth, for the nobility of her aspect, and for the extraordinary gifts of nature and furthermore so skilled in portraying the human features, as to show that no one has been her equal in her own time, in the year 1632.'[72]

A Genoese Merchant: Desiderio Segno

Another member of the Genoese community in Palermo, closely associated with Orazio Lomellini, Sofonisba's husband, was Desiderio Segno. His father, Giovan Agostino Segno, had moved from the small town of Signo on the Ligurian coast to Palermo and was already documented there by 1611, as one of the *rettori* of San Giorgio dei Genovesi.[73] The family acquired a chapel in the north transept of San Giorgio (fig. 19), which had been decorated with an altarpiece of the *Baptism of Christ* by Jacopo Palma il Giovane, commissioned by the Genoese community (this was moved to another chapel in the church in the eighteenth century and substituted with a Crucifix).[74] An inscription over the arch of the chapel records the dedication by Giovan Agostino Segno and the date 1621. Another inscription, originally on the step in front of the altar, recorded Giovan Agostino's death in 1620, and how the tomb had been commissioned by his widow and by his son.[75] Desiderio's mother was Camilla Ventimiglia, who was related to Carlo Maria Ventimiglia, the 'principe' of the Accademia dei Riaccesi.[76]

Segno's family business was one of the most important mercantile enterprises in Palermo in the early seventeenth century. Giovan Agostino had worked with his two sons, Desiderio and Giovan Francesco, but after the latter's death in 1617, Desiderio was joined

20 | Ruins of the castle, Salaparuta

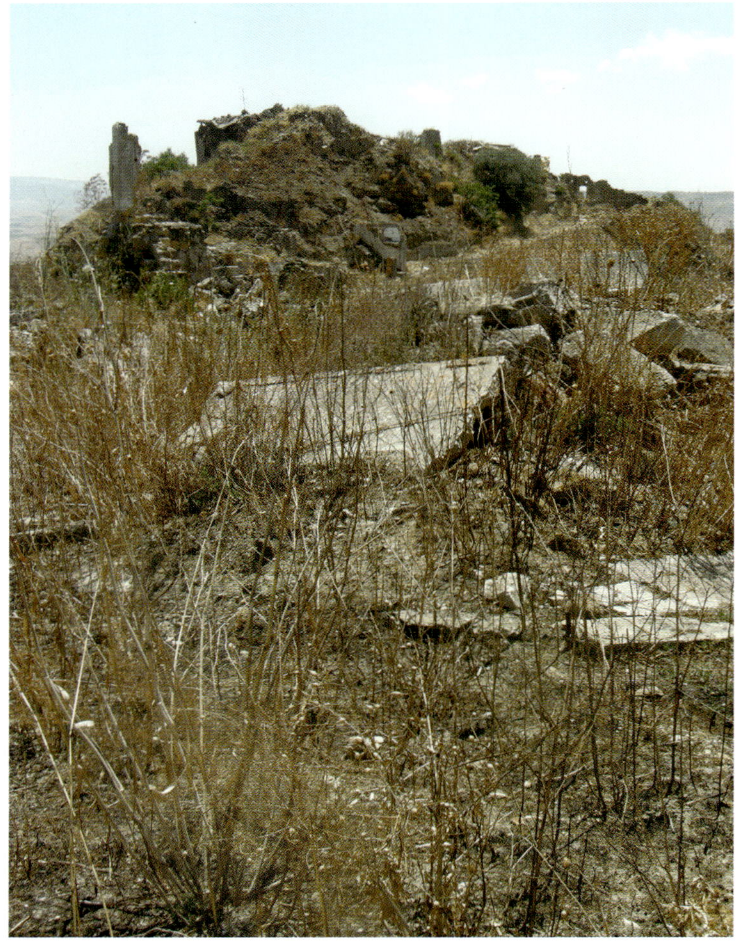

in the business by Giovan Agostino Arata, who had married Virginia, his sister.[77] Desiderio was a prominent member of the Genoese community and his brother-in-law was in business with Cardinal Giannettino Doria.[78] From 1615, Segno had been a *massaro* of the Genoese community, together with Orazio Lomellini, and between November 1623 and December 1624, in the period when Van Dyck first arrived in Palermo, he had been *console* of the community. The two *massari* during that time were Orazio Lomellini and Giovan Agostino Arata.[79] Segno owned a palace in the town of Salaparuta (fig. 20) where he lived with his wife, Flavia Tortorici, a young son and two girls, and his brother-in-law. He died in December 1630 in Salaparuta, and was buried at San Giorgio dei Genovesi.[80]

The *post-mortem* inventory of Segno's possessions, of 24 December 1630, reveals that he had been portrayed by Van Dyck.[81] One of the items listed in the document is 'a portrait of the deceased Signor Desiderio, by Anthony van Dyck, with a black frame', and this has been reasonably identified with the portrait now in the Liechtenstein Collection (cat. 8).[82] Displayed in the collection were three more paintings by Van Dyck: 'a painting of Saint Rosalia in glory, by Anthony van Dyck, with a black frame' identifiable with the *Saint Rosalia* in the Metropolitan Museum (cat. 16), 'a painting of a deposition from the cross, by the same, with a frame as above' and 'a painting with a head who yawns, by the same Van Dyck, with a black and gold frame', both now lost.[83] Segno's collection of paintings was not large but, apart from four paintings by Van Dyck, it included pictures by significant artists: he owned a *Bath of Nymphs* painted on stone by Luca Cambiaso, and a portrait by Sofonisba Anguissola of her father Amilcare – possibly a gift by the painter to Desiderio.[84]

Interesting links between Segno and another painting that Van Dyck made in Sicily are known from another document, of 22 April 1626. On that date, Segno declared that he was holding a group of five paintings as security against 80 *onze* ('*tenet loco pignoris unciarum octaginta*'), which he had lent to Fabrizio Valguarnera on 6 May 1624.[85] Valguarnera's wife, Giovanna, promised to pay within the next month so that Segno would return the five pictures. Four were said to be by Titian and were Old Testament scenes from the life of Moses: *Pharaoh Submerged in the Red Sea*, the *Fall of Manna*, *Moses Striking the Rock* and the *Golden Calf*. The fifth painting was a *Stoning of Saint Stephen* by Van Dyck.[86] It has been suggested that Valguarnera's picture may have been a copy of Van Dyck's canvas now at Tatton Park (cat. 9), but it is likely that it could have been the original.[87]

'*Dottore in Palermo*': Fabrizio Valguarnera

The name of Fabrizio Valguarnera, the man who owed Desiderio Segno 80 *onze* and had left him five paintings as security, including the *Stoning of Saint Stephen* by Van Dyck, appears on the second page of the artist's *Italian Sketchbook* (fig. 21 and cat. 5). Inscribed in Van Dyck's own hand, next to some sketches is '*Don Fabricio Malguarnero [sic] Dottore in Palermo*'.[88] Van Dyck must have been given Valguarnera's name as someone he should meet in Palermo and took note of it. Both Rubens and Cornelis de Wael knew Valguarnera and it is likely that it was one of them who made the introduc-

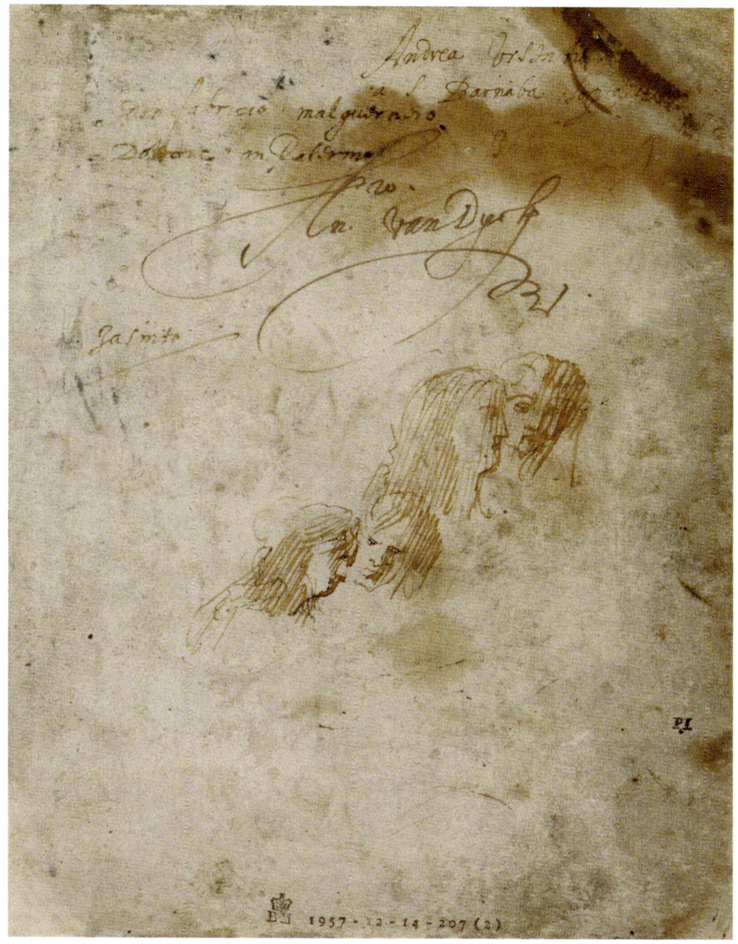

21 | Sir Anthony van Dyck,
Italian Sketchbook – Fabrizio Valguarnera's name
The British Museum, London, fol. 2r

tion.[89] Van Dyck must have known little about Valguarnera at the time, but he was one of the most fascinating characters in the Italian world of the first half of the seventeenth century. He has been aptly described as belonging to 'that race of adventurers that a century later Italy would bestow upon Europe: Casanovas and Cagliostros', between 'the murky shades of diamond smuggler, almost a sort of devilish *ante litteram* Count of Cagliostro, and those of the adventurer-connoisseur and merchant-amateur'.[90]

Valguarnera described himself as 'from Palermo', but his exact origins are unclear.[91] He was possibly the illegitimate son of a member of the aristocratic Valguarnera family; after his death in Rome, his mother Beatrice appeared in front of a notary on 15 April 1632 to establish her identity and to give the priest Carlo Venezia power of attorney to take over her son's properties in Rome.[92] Valguarnera is documented as buying a carriage in Palermo in May 1620, and in September 1625 he married Giovanna Gaeta, widow of Paolo de Diana.[93] Between 1628 and 1629 he travelled to Madrid, where he joined his uncle Mariano Valguarnera, who was chaplain to King Philip IV.[94] Valguarnera must have been knowledgeable about art: he described himself as 'having an understanding of, and pleasure in, painting, that is not that I paint, but I have knowledge and taste for good pictures', and he was referred to by others as being an expert ('*prattico di Pitture*').[95]

The agreement of 22 April 1626 between Valguarnera, his wife Giovanna, and Desiderio Segno about the loan and the five paintings being held as security (including Van Dyck's *Stoning of Saint Stephen*) should not appear unusual if it was not for a previous document of 3 February 1623 which, in the light also of later events in Valguarnera's life, casts a shadow on the deal. Valguarnera had commissioned, a year before the loan from Segno (in May 1624), copies of four paintings from the Flemish artist Hieronymus Gerards.[96] These were four Old Testament scenes representing the *Fall of Manna*, *Moses Striking the Rock*, the *Pharaoh Submerged in the Red Sea* and the *Golden Calf* – surely the same paintings described as being by Titian in the 1626 document. The suspicion arises that Valguarnera had given Segno as security against the loan, not four paintings by Titian, but four copies of them by Gerards.[97] This is impossible to prove but the later infamous case of Valguarnera's involvement in diamond smuggling is worth recalling in detail, as the final chapter of his criminal activity that surely must have had its seeds already in Palermo in the 1620s.

On 20 June 1631, Rubens wrote to Valguarnera: he was planning to paint an *Adoration of the Magi* for him, but had not heard from him and was not sure if 'you are in Naples or in Palermo, or in another place; however I hope that this letter will reach you as I know that gentlemen like you are known everywhere'.[98] Apparently Rubens had met Valguarnera in Madrid and had been cured of gout by him. Two months earlier, on 20 April, Cornelis de Wael had also written from Genoa to Valguarnera. It seems that Valguarnera had been in touch with Van Dyck, by then back in Antwerp, about a further commission; De Wael wanted to inform Valguarnera that the painting was almost finished and Van Dyck was going to send it to Palermo as soon as possible, and then enquired about a portrait by Titian.[99] Rubens, Van Dyck and De Wael did not know that, as they were writing to Palermo and looking for Valguarnera, their patron

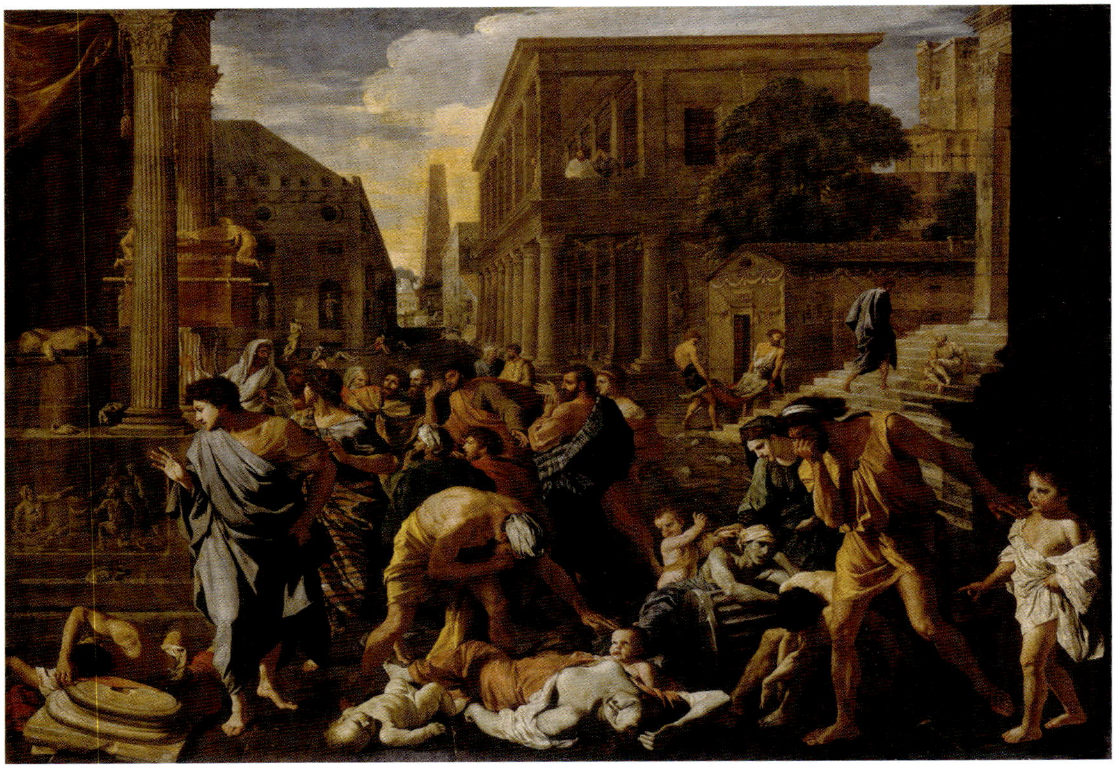

22 | Nicolas Poussin,
The Plague at Ashdod
Musée du Louvre, Paris

was involved in one of the most intriguing criminal trials of the seventeenth century.[100] On 12 July 1631 the office of the Governor of Rome, and the police, were informed by three Flemish merchants in Madrid – Balthasare and Ferdinando de Groote and Paulo Sonnio – that a significant number of uncut diamonds, belonging to them, had been stolen between October and November 1629. The stones had arrived in Lisbon from the Indies and the merchants had them sent with a courier over the mountains to Madrid; there they were received by a young Portuguese man, Manuel Alvares Carapeto, who was their cashier. Once delivered, the diamonds were supposed to be divided between the three merchants who had acquired them, but Manuel disappeared in Madrid with the diamonds. The merchants knew Valguarnera, and knew that he was close to Manuel's wife Giovanna (they did not know, however, that the two were probably having an affair), so they asked him to investigate and retrieve the diamonds. Needless to say, Valguarnera had also disappeared. The merchants told the Roman police that they had already spent thousands of *scudi* trying to locate the thieves over the past two years in Barcelona, Seville, Palermo, Messina and other Italian cities. By this point they were looking principally for Valguarnera, as they concluded that he would have been easier to identify, as Manuel may have changed his name and it was more difficult for a nobleman to do so, and also because they assumed that by now Valguarnera, probably following the 'inspiration of the Devil' must have already killed Manuel.[101] The merchants told the police that Valguarnera 'has a degree in law, he is a mathematician, and is also an expert in medicine, and has healed Rubens from gout'.[102] They also suggested that Cornelis de Wael in Genoa might have known his whereabouts; they had heard that Valguarnera was in Rome and, having had the diamonds cut, was buying paintings with them. They demanded that Valguarnera should be arrested, and on that same day he was found in a house near the church of San Silvestro and brought with his belongings to the prison of Tor di Nona.

The trial soon began. In the early days of August 1631 Valguarnera started to recount his version of the events. Manuel had told him about the theft and he had reached him in Bayonne, in France, in March 1630; together they travelled to Toulouse, Lyons, Orange and Toulon and in June they reached Genoa. Manuel had been disposing of the diamonds '*alla gagliarda*' and had been spending them on 'clothes and whores'.[103] Valguarnera confessed that during the trip 'there came to me certain temptations of the Devil… to kill this Manuel, or rather to have him killed, so that all the said diamonds would remain for me, and one evening, that I remember was a Tuesday, I believe it was in the month of June of last year [1630], while we were travelling, it was the vigil of the Madonna di Costantinopoli, there came to me in the night a great temptation to kill the said Manuel, wherefore I (addressed) myself to the Madonna, praying to her to lift these temptations from me, and in the night I felt myself awaken, and it seemed to me that I heard the voice of a woman who said, take care what you do, and I think that this was in the lazaret of Genoa or another place near-by; I hearing thus was stirred, believing that this was the Madonna, and I awoke, and embraced the said Manuel, who was sleeping with me, and he said to me what was the matter, and I said to him that it was nothing, and gave

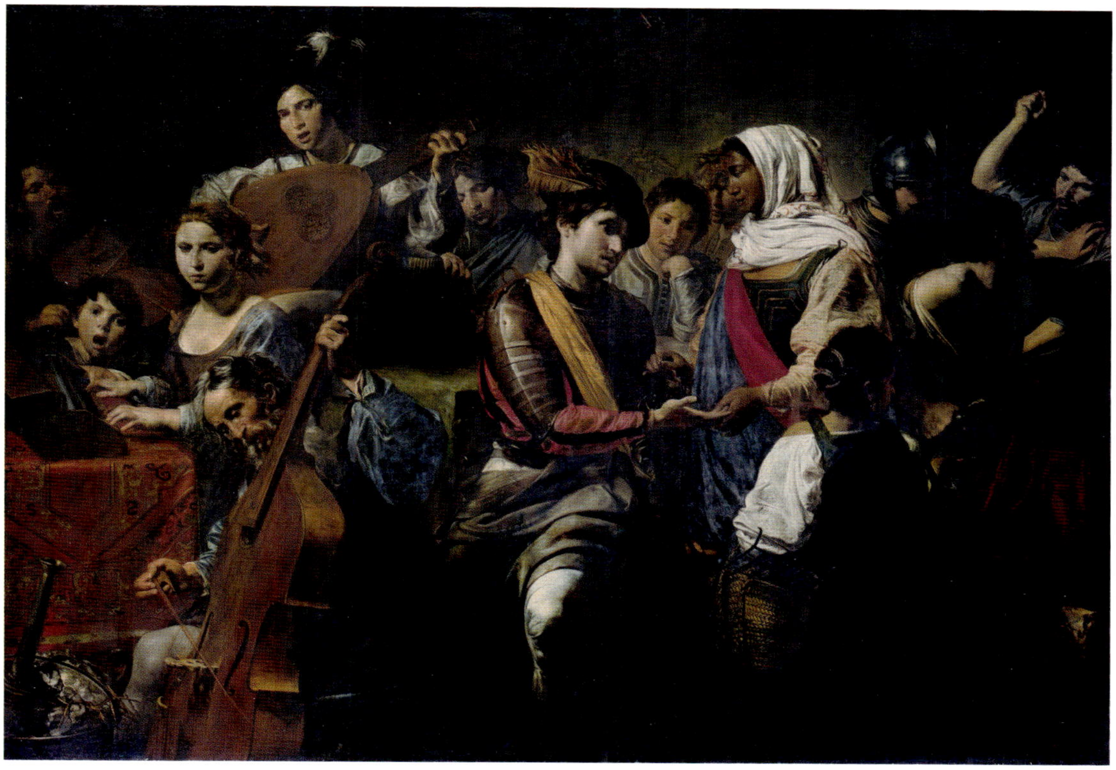

23 | Valentin de Boulogne,
Concert with a Gipsy Fortune Teller
Liechtenstein. The Princely Collections, Vaduz-Vienna

his life in sacrifice to the Madonna di Costantinopoli, and undertook as a devotion always to fast on her festival, and to have a mass said every Tuesday.'[104] They proceeded south to Leghorn, Naples and arrived in Rome in the autumn, with Manuel still using the diamonds. By Christmas Valguarnera claimed to have convinced Manuel to travel back to Spain and return what was left of the spoils of their theft. Manuel departed with thirteen bags of diamonds under a false name, and Valguarnera established himself in Rome under the name of '*Antonio Siciliano*'. He maintained he never heard from Manuel again except for one letter he received from him from Genoa. Notwithstanding his supposed good intentions, Valguarnera must have kept with him a significant number of diamonds, as he proceeded to exchange diamonds for paintings over the next six months in Rome.

A clearer sense of Valguarnera's art dealing emerges from the trial documents. On 10 June 1631 Valguarnera lent a group of paintings for a public exhibition at Santa Maria di Costantinopoli – the church of the Sicilian community in Rome – as thanksgiving for his Genoese vision and for having spared Manuel's life.[105] When Valguarnera was arrested in July, thirty-seven paintings were found in his house, together with diamonds. He was said to have brought paintings with him from Palermo to Madrid in 1628 (possibly including Van Dyck's *Stoning of Saint Stephen*; see cat. 9), and had sold them once in Spain. He had subsequently bought more pictures and commissioned others. The Roman judges called many art dealers and painters to the stand in July 1631. The dealer Ferrante Carlo admitted to having sold paintings – a *Madonna* by Ludovico Carracci, a *Portrait of Bembo* by Titian, a *Charity* that was either by Dosso Dossi or by Guido Reni, a *Madonna* probably by Correggio and other works – in exchange for diamonds. Another dealer, Giovan Stefano Roccatagliata, had also sold him paintings for diamonds, including pictures by Annibale Carracci, Poussin and Valentin de Boulogne. But it turned out that Valguarnera had also gone directly to the painters and commissioned works by them. Both Valentin and Giovanni Lanfranco were paid in diamonds; Turchi had not finished his painting for Valguarnera by the time he was arrested, and Poussin claimed he was paid in *scudi*, even though Lanfranco testified that he had heard that Poussin too had been given diamonds. It seems likely that the two paintings commissioned from Rubens and Van Dyck, and to which the letters of April and June 1631 refer to, were also part of Valguarnera's plan to 'invest' the diamonds he had stolen. As both artists were abroad, the Roman judges never questioned them and their names do not appear in the court proceedings, but the fact that both painters were at work for Valguarnera in 1631 suggests that the enterprise of commissioning pictures was on an international scale.

It is apparent that Valguarnera was buying paintings using the diamonds he had stolen. It is not clear, however, which of these pictures were shown at Santa Maria di Costantinopoli – if the exhibition ever happened at all. Joachim von Sandrart, in the autobiography that precedes the main body of his *Teutsche Academie* (published in Nuremberg in 1675), records that he moved to Rome and 'as soon as two pieces by his hand had seen the day, he was counted among those most famous painters in Italy who were to make twelve pieces for the

King of Spain, of like size after life; he then so successfully completed his work that it was esteemed as one of the best by cardinals, dukes, princes, and dilettanti in Rome, when, on the feast day of Our Lady of Constantinople, they were exhibited in the course of the procession'.[106] Sandrart claimed to have painted a *Death of Seneca* as part of this group of pictures, and the other eleven were *The Abduction of Helen* by Guido Reni, *The Death of Dido* by Guercino, *The Rape of the Sabine Women* by Pietro da Cortona, the *Five Senses* by Valentin, *Divine Wisdom* by Andrea Sacchi, *Diana, Callisto and Acteon* by Lanfranco, *The Hunt of Diana* by Domenichino, *The Plague at Ashdod* by Poussin, two paintings of unknown subjects by Cavalier d'Arpino and Massimo Stanzione that were not finished in time for the exhibition, and one by Orazio Gentileschi that he had kept in England with him. Sandrart repeated the story in the Latin edition of his book in 1683, but when discussing Poussin's *Plague at Ashdod* (fig. 22) he reported that 'it had been executed, six feet wide and four high, with incomparable judgment, for a certain Sicilian art-lover whose name was Antonio. In as much as Antonio was afterwards thrown into prison for debts and there died, this picture was sold at public auction to a certain nobleman of Pozzuoli for one thousand silver crowns'.[107] The relationship between the group of pictures for the King of Spain and Valguarnera's own, and their exhibition in Rome in 1631 is confused in Sandrart's accounts. The group of paintings must have been of varying quality. The Reni and Guercino were destined for Spain, but the other ten had no link to the king. Both the Domenichino and Pietro da Cortona paintings must have been copies of the famous pictures in the Borghese and Sacchetti collections; Sacchi's *Divine Wisdom* was a fresco in the Barberini Palace, so Sandrart must have been referring to a subsequent version of it on canvas. This was not a specifically designed 'set' of paintings for the King of Spain, as Sandrart implied, but a combination of works commissioned from Spain and others that belonged to Valguarnera. A list of Valguarnera's goods of 21 July 1631 includes the *Plague at Ashdod* and a *Triumph of Flora* by Poussin, the *Rape of the Sabine Women* by Pietro da Cortona, and Valentin's *Concert with a Gipsy Fortune Teller* (fig. 23).[108] Interestingly, among the paintings there was also a copy of Poussin's *Plague* by Angelo Caroselli, which we know Valguarnera had paid for.[109] Once again, he owned originals and copies of the same picture, possibly with a view to more dishonest activities. The *Plague*, with its early morning fearful vision of destruction and the dying groups of Philistines, must have resonated with Valguarnera who, in 1624, was in Palermo and would have witnessed the plague there.

On Christmas Day 1631 Valguarnera signed his will in the prison of Tor di Nona. He asked to be buried in Santa Maria di Costantinopoli and left his money to 'S.r Emanuele Alberto Scarapeto di Portugallo della Città di Elbes', his companion in crime, Manuel.[110] A few days later, on 2 January 1632, it was recorded that 'this morning Fabrizio Valguarnera died, who found himself prisoner in Tor di Nona on the charge of the theft of diamonds after having been sick with fever many days'.[111] It is unclear if he was poisoned, or the cause of his death was natural. With his disappearance, however, the trial stopped, and there is no further news of the diamonds, Manuel or the fate of the paintings. By 1635 the Valguarnera family had taken possession of his belongings.[112] As Van Dyck was writing down Valguarnera's name in his sketchbook, and as he was painting the *Stoning of Saint Stephen* for him while in Sicily, he could not have imagined that he was dealing with the future author of one of the most infamous art-related heists of the seventeenth century.

Saint Rosalia and the Plague

Van Dyck's sojourn in Palermo coincided with the city's nascent cult of Saint Rosalia, which had begun with the finding of her relics in 1624. Rosalia lived between 1130 and 1170, and was said to have been the daughter of a certain Sinibaldo, a nobleman from Palermo at the court of King Roger.[113] She lived in isolation as a hermit first in a cave at the Quisquina (fig. 24), in the mountainous region north of Agrigento, and then outside Palermo on the Monte Pellegrino. She may have been a Basilian nun at the convent next to Santa Maria dell'Ammiraglio (the so-called Martorana), and the first image of her is from an icon from that convent (fig. 25), where she appears together with three other saints, Oliva, Elia and Venera.[114] Most of her life, however, was spent in a cave on the Monte Pellegrino, where she was thought to have died. A group of Franciscan hermits was established on the Monte Pellegrino from at least the mid-sixteenth century, and they were known as the Romiti di Monte Pellegrino.

Rosalia had already been invoked as a saintly intercessor against the plague in 1494 and in 1530.[115] As the plague hit Palermo during the summer of 1624, the hermits started to look for the bones of Saint Rosalia on the Monte Pellegrino. This interest in relics of earlier saints had been particularly fashionable in Rome in recent years, particularly around the Jubilee of 1600.[116] On 15 July 1624, a few days after Van Dyck's visit to Sofonisba Anguissola, the saint's relics were found in a cave on the Monte Pellegrino by a lone hunter.[117] On 30 November, Archbishop Giannettino Doria created a commission to examine the bones and establish their authenticity as relics. The group of experts, which included Giovan Francesco Fiocchetto, Emanuele Filiberto's physician, concluded between 15 and 18 February 1625 that the bones were indeed those of a woman, and possibly of more than one individual.[118] On 22 February the relics were officially declared genuine by Doria, and the Senate stipulated that chapels in the Cathedral and on the Monte Pellegrino should be dedicated to Rosalia.[119] The bones were then placed in a silver and crystal reliquary (fig. 26), commissioned by Nicola Placito and Giacomo Agliata on behalf of the Senate on 3 March 1625, and made by a team of artists that included Giancola Viviano, Apollonio Mancuso, Francesco Licco, Desiderio Pillitteri and Giovanni Di Pietro.[120] On 15 August Rosalia was proclaimed patron saint of Palermo. The city already had four female patron saints – Christina, Ninfa, Oliva and Agatha – but immediately Rosalia, known affectionately as the *santuzza*, took over as the principal saint in Palermo.

From the moment Rosalia's bones were found, the relics were used by the Archbishop of Palermo to combat the plague that was ravaging the city. Since a few people had been miraculously healed by the relics, Giannettino Doria ordered that the bones should be processed through the city to stop the spread of the infection.[121] On 6 June 1625, Doria issued an edict stating that 'even though it is to be hoped in the liberation from the contagious disease through the intercession of glorious Saint Rosalia, patron and citizen of this city, however, the human instruments and industry should not be set aside'.[122] The body of Saint Rosalia was exhibited in the Cathedral for eight days that summer, and people from the different quarters of the city were allowed to visit the relics on specific days of the week. As the plague seemed to diminish by September, Doria issued a further edict, and he established the saint's feast day on 4 September.[123] However, the fight against the plague was a long and difficult one. By 6 January 1626, Doria was still issuing rules and policies against the plague in the city. Notwithstanding Rosalia's miraculous intervention, Doria had set a series of strict regulations trying to prevent the plague from spreading further. He ordered the inhabitants of Palermo to deliver any infected or suspect object to the appropriate authority to avoid being excommunicated.[124] After the term of eight days had expired, anyone who had not complied with this would be excommunicated, and 'each one of these people will be cursed in eating and drinking, in being awake, and in sleeping, in raising from their beds, in walking, in living and in dying; the Devil will be next to them, and in the time of Judgment, they will be condemned: their days will be few and bad, their goods and belongings will be given to foreigners, their children will be needy orphans; their houses and dwellings burnt, they will be hated to the extent that they will not find a single person who will feel

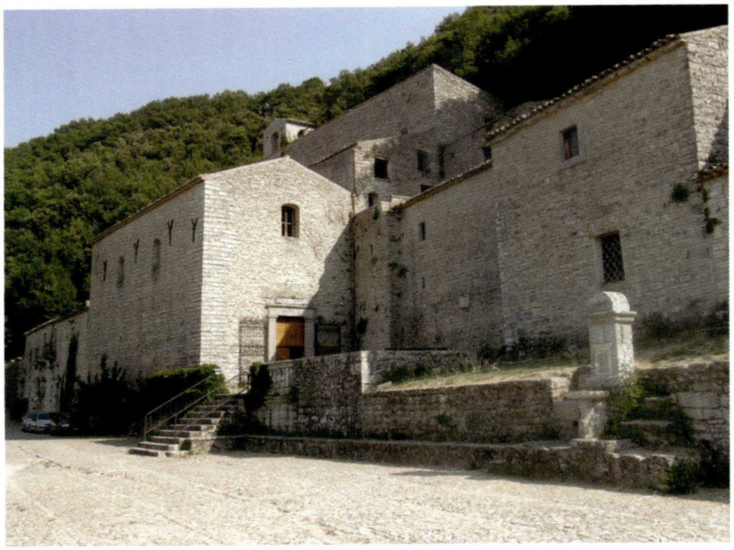

24 | Quisquina, Eremo of Saint Rosalia

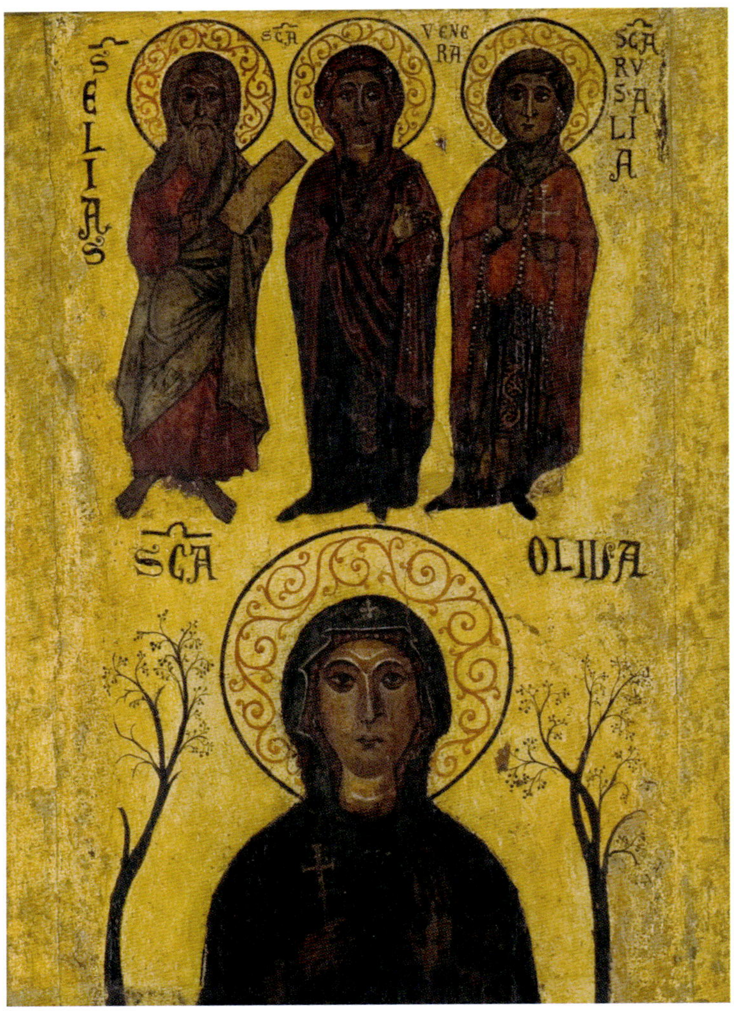

25 | Anonymous, *Saints Oliva, Elia, Venera and Rosalia*
Museo Diocesano, Palermo

sorry for them or their progeny; their evil will constantly be in front of God, the bread, the wine, the meat, the fish and all that they will eat and drink will be cursed; the clothes they will wear, and the bed in which they shall sleep will be cursed, with every curse of the Old and New Testament; they will be cursed with Lucifer, and Judas and all the Devils in hell, who will accompany them'.[125] All priests were ordered not to give these people the absolution from confession and the citizens of Palermo were exhorted to pray that no one would die this way.

Saint Rosalia was seen as a protector of the city from the early days of the plague in the summer of 1624 until its end in 1626. When Emanuele Filiberto was taken ill, an image of the saint, probably derived from the Martorana icon (fig. 25), was taken in procession by the Jesuits on 1 August 1624. The painting is lost, but a canvas by Vito D'Anna in the church of the Gesù may be a copy of this image.[126] The first feast (known as *festino*) dedicated to Saint Rosalia took place in July 1625, the relics of the saint were paraded through the city, and different communities in the city built triumphal arches along the route.[127] By this date, the iconography of Rosalia was being established by artists in Palermo – Van Dyck above all. Not many images of the saint existed before 1624, and a few examples survive by Sicilian artists such as Tommaso da Vigilia, Francesco Traini, Domenico Gagini and Antonello Crescenzio.[128] As recently argued, the first documented image of Saint Rosalia in 1624 was produced by Vincenzo La Barbera (cat. 11), probably commissioned by the Senate; it is likely that this painting was brought in procession across the city on 4 September 1624.[129] The artist's daughter was said to have been healed through the miraculous intercession of the saint.[130] La Barbera showed Rosalia praying for the city ravaged by the plague, and a second painting by him, in the church of Sant'Anna, represents a similar subject (fig. 27).

Van Dyck created the standard image of Saint Rosalia as it is still known in Sicily. In his paintings the saint is a young and beautiful woman with flowing blonde hair, dressed in a brown monastic dress. Her attributes are roses (a reference to her name) and lilies, and a skull often accompanied by a book. The skull may have been a direct reference to the relics that were found on the Monte

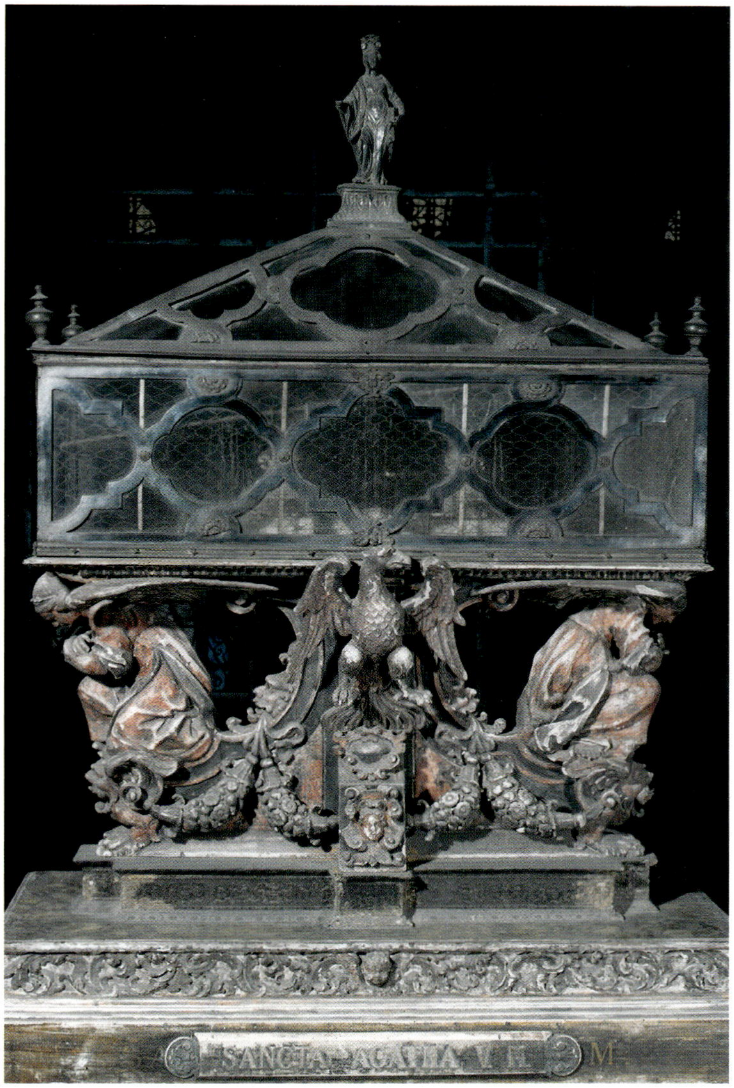

26 | Giancola Viviano, Apollonio Mancuso, Francesco Licco, Desiderio Pillitteri, Giovanni Di Pietro, *First Reliquary Urn of Saint Rosalia*
Cathedral, Palermo

Pellegrino in the summer of 1624, but may also have been more generally linked to the iconography of hermit saints. Following the example of La Barbera's paintings (cat. 11 and fig. 27), Van Dyck also usually set the figure of the saint within a view of Palermo to stress the close connection between Rosalia and her city. At least five images of Saint Rosalia by Van Dyck survive, and more might have been painted. There seem to have been two predominant ways in which the saint was depicted: praying for the city from her cave on Monte Pellegrino, in an iconographical type that was close to representations of hermit saints like the Magdalene, Saint Francis of Assisi and Saint Jerome (cats. 12–14); and another kind in which Rosalia appeared triumphant and in glory, closer to images of the Virgin's Assumption (cat. 16). Charles Sterling in 1939 wrote that 'it would no doubt be presumptuous, in the total absence of any document, to try to establish a chronological estimate of the different versions of St. Rosalie that Van Dyck produced in Palermo.'[131] He, however, proposed that most of them were made or at least begun in Palermo, with the exception of the canvas in Ponce (cat. 12), which he believed was painted after the artist returned to Antwerp. More recently it has been suggested that all of the paintings of Saint Rosalia were produced in Sicily, most likely between the procession in which La Barbera's painting (cat. 11) was exhibited in September 1624, and September 1625 when Van Dyck left Sicily.[132] Gauvin Alexander Bailey, in his 2005 study on Van Dyck's paintings of Saint Rosalia, put forward a new chronology, which is so far the most reasonable and convincing.[133] For Bailey, Van Dyck's first image of Rosalia was the one closest to La Barbera's example (cat. 11), the Ponce canvas (cat. 12), which is almost identical in subject to the canvas by the Sicilian artist.[134] This picture was followed by the other paintings of the saint as a hermit interceding for Palermo, now in London (cat. 13) and Houston (cat. 14).[135] The painting *Saint Rosalia in Glory Interceding for Palermo*, in New York (cat. 16), was likely the last one to be painted by Van Dyck in Palermo. A further canvas, attributed to Van Dyck, and possibly from his Sicilian period is *The Virgin Presenting Saint Rosalia to the Trinity* in the Alte Pinakothek in Munich (114 x 88 cm – fig. 28). The poor condition of the painting makes a firm attribution to the artist difficult, but it is likely that this picture may have been produced in Palermo.[136] A copy of it survives in a private collection in Palermo, and Willem Walsgart's altarpiece with *Saint Rosalia Interceding for the Town of Ciminna* in the Chiesa Madre of Ciminna, near Palermo, derives directly from the Munich painting.[137]

Around the same time that Van Dyck was producing his paintings of Rosalia, between 1624 and 1625, another artist, the Tuscan sculptor Gregorio Tedeschi, was at work on an important image of the saint. He had been given public commissions in the city, such as the sculpture of *Spring* for the Quattro Canti, in 1620–24 (in 1630 he also made the statue of *Saint Christina* for the same location), and the altar of Saint Francis Xavier (*c.* 1622) for the Jesuit church in Palermo.[138] The cave where the saint's human remains were found (fig. 29) had become an important site of pilgrimage, promoted by

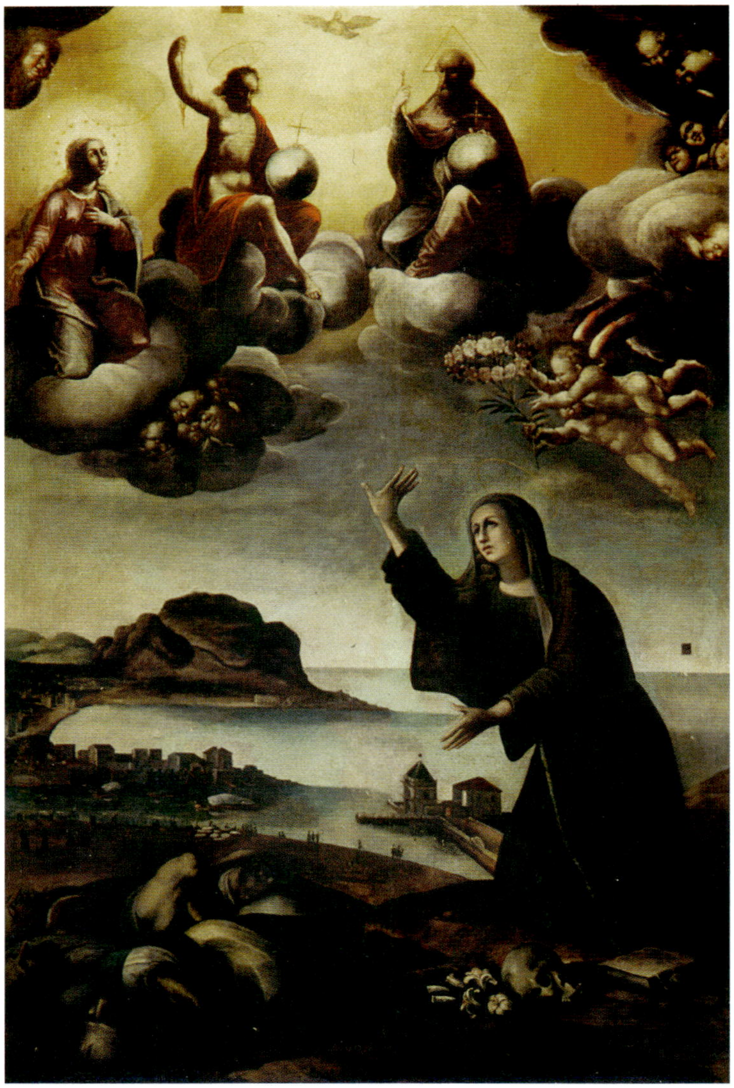

27 | Vincenzo La Barbera, *Saint Rosalia Interceding for Palermo*
Sant'Anna la Misericordia, Palermo

the Archbishop and the city. It was the Senate, who had commissioned La Barbera's image of Rosalia (cat. 11), who also asked Tedeschi to produce a recumbent statue in Carrara marble of the dying saint for the cave (fig. 30). The work, carved in 1625, is in fact, as noted by Bailey in 2005, the first sculpture of a saint lying down in agony (or ecstasy) in the Baroque era, long before Giovan Lorenzo Bernini.[139]

Around 1625 the cult of Rosalia developed rapidly. By being in Palermo, Van Dyck knew the public commissions to local artists, such as La Barbera, and foreign ones, like Tedeschi. Even though in the immediate aftermath of the finding of the relics he did not receive any official commissions, and it is likely that most of his paintings of Saint Rosalia were produced for local private patrons, he managed, starting from La Barbera's prototype, to invent and promote the most influential and lasting image of Rosalia. As Charles Sterling noted, 'Van Dyck's is the ideal saint of the Counter-Reformation in its most universal prestige; her charm is equally for the aristocrat and for the man of the people.'[140]

Van Dyck's Sicilian Paintings

Only about ten paintings survive from Van Dyck's Sicilian period, but many more are documented in Sicilian seventeenth-century inventories. Desiderio Segno, for example, owned not only his portrait by Van Dyck (cat. 8) and a *Saint Rosalia* (cat. 16), but also two paintings that are now lost, a *Deposition* and a picture of a 'yawning head' ('*una testa che badiglia*').[141]

The will of Simone Sitaiolo of 26 February 1632 mentions a portrait of him and four works 'painted by the hand of Anthony Van Dyck, the Fleming'.[142] The subsequent inventory of Sitaiolo's possessions, of 20 March 1632, lists the four other paintings by Van Dyck: a *Satyr*, a large *Saint John* (see cat. 10), a *Saint Rosalia*, and a *Virgin and Child with Saint Rosalia and Saint John*.[143] On 24 April of that year, don Gaspare Ventimiglia took in custody, on behalf of Sitaiolo's heirs, the portrait, two of the Van Dycks (the *Saint Rosalia* and the *Satyr*), a *Martyrdom of Saint Placidus* (the author is not mentioned) and a miniature of the *Nativity*, possibly by Castello; all the other paintings were probably sold.[144]

28 | Attributed to Anthony van Dyck,
The Virgin Presenting Saint Rosalia to the Trinity
Bayerische Staatsgemäldesammlungen, Alte Pinakothek, Munich

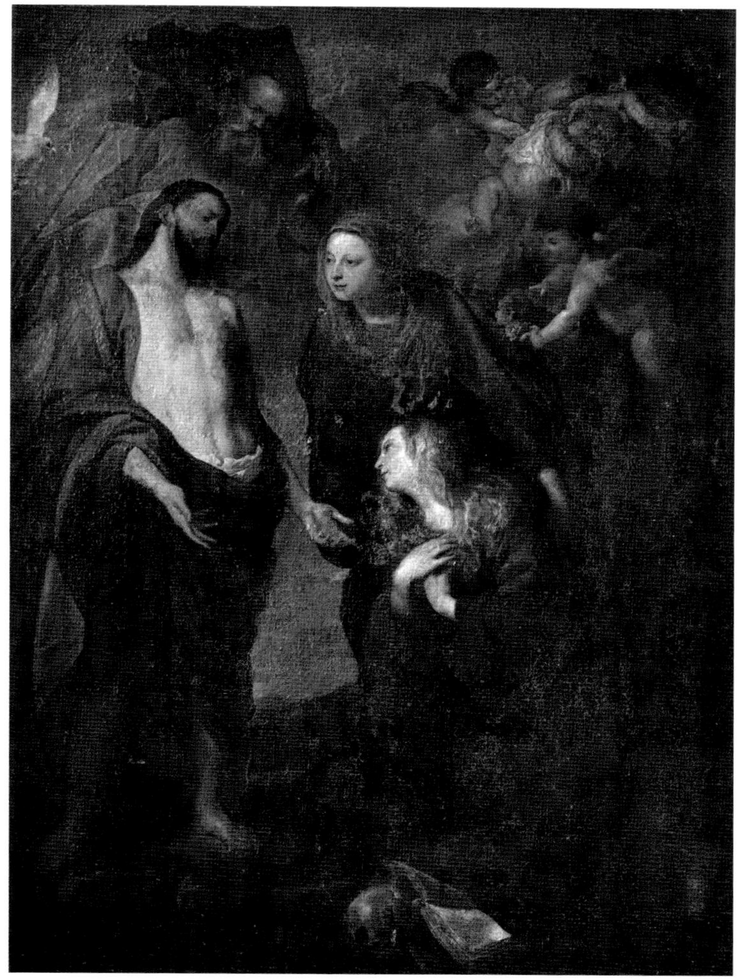

Don Tommaso Joppolo, Maestro Segreto del Regno from 1628, had a significant collection of about 180 paintings, which included works by Titian, Tintoretto, Ribera, Strozzi, Bassano and Manfredi. His inventory of 1639 listed six paintings by Van Dyck: a *Magdalene*, a *Saint Anthony*, a 'Virgin with the Child holding his crown in his hand', a *Deposition with the Virgin, Saint John and the Magdalene* (which may have been the same painting that had belonged to Segno), a *Madonna of the Rosary with Various Figures* (possibly a sketch or replica of Van Dyck's altarpiece), and a 'Virgin holding the Child in her arms'.[145]

The '*cappellano*' of the Cathedral, don Marco Gezio, owned a *Saint Rosalia*, 'measuring five palmi by four', which appears in his 1658 inventory.[146] Cristoforo Papè, a Flemish collector in Palermo, in 1666, had a large *Ecce Homo*, a *Madonna within a Garland of Roses* and a copy of the *Madonna of the Rosary*.[147] Antonio Lucchese del Campo e Jeijsen, Prince of Campofranco, left in his will of 5 December 1651 to his aunt, Antonia Bologna Ventimiglia, Marchesa di Altavilla, 'a painting of the Virgin and Child by Van Dyck' and to the '*procuratore*' don Pietro Gaudiuso 'a painting of Our Lady of Mercy by Van Dyck'.[148]

Don Antonio Ruffo, who bought Desiderio Segno's *Saint Rosalia* (cat. 16) in Palermo, in 1648, owned also two other paintings attributed to Van Dyck. Ruffo's expense book, compiled before 1655, records the acquisition of a 'head of a satyr by Van Dyck' on paper.[149] Subsequent inventories of the Ruffo family – of 1 January 1652, 1 January 1668 and of 1677 – list the *Saint Rosalia* and the *Head of a Satyr* and a third painting, a portrait bought for 24 *onze*. The portrait is identified as that of a painter ('*pittore*') in the 1652 inventory, but the word is subsequently corrected as 'doctor' ('*dottore*'), and it is specified that the sitter is without a hat and holding a book in his hand ('*scoperto che tiene un libro in mano*').[150]

That Van Dyck produced oil sketches on paper while in Palermo is proved by the lawsuit of September 1625 against his '*creato*', Domenico Martinetto, who had stolen several works on paper from his master's workshop. It seems, however, that some of these objects were collected in Sicily. Not only Antonio Ruffo owned the *Head of a Satyr* on paper but also, by 1666, the painter Filippo Fini owned various 'oil sketches on paper by Van Dyck'.[151]

Copies after paintings by Van Dyck were also produced in Sicily in the seventeenth century and are documented in contemporary inventories. On 18 June 1626, Giovanni Battista Grasso, a painter from Messina, signed a contract to produce a 'Saint Rosalia copied from Anthony Van Dyck, with the angels in glory, similar to the one copied from Anthony Van Dyck'.[152] In 1667 Giuseppe Corrado sold to the Genoese don Fabrizio Castelli two copies after Van Dyck, an unfinished *Annunciation* and a 'Madonna with Saint Rosalia and other figures'.[153] The inventory of 8 August 1682 of the paintings of don Vincenzo Gallego, Principe di Militello, lists an 'Ecce Homo copied from Van Dyck'.[154]

The *Madonna of the Rosary*

Van Dyck's production of portraits of prominent Sicilians, and of devotional images, mainly centred around the figure of Saint Rosalia, placed him in the position to receive the most prestigious commission of his Sicilian years, that for a large public altarpiece. The

29 | Cave of Saint Rosalia from G. Cascini, *Di Santa Rosalia, romita palermitana, palesata con libri tre* (Palermo 1651)
Biblioteca centrale della Regione siciliana 'Alberto Bombace', Palermo

30 | Gregorio Tedeschi, *Saint Rosalia*
Santuario di Monte Pellegrino, Palermo

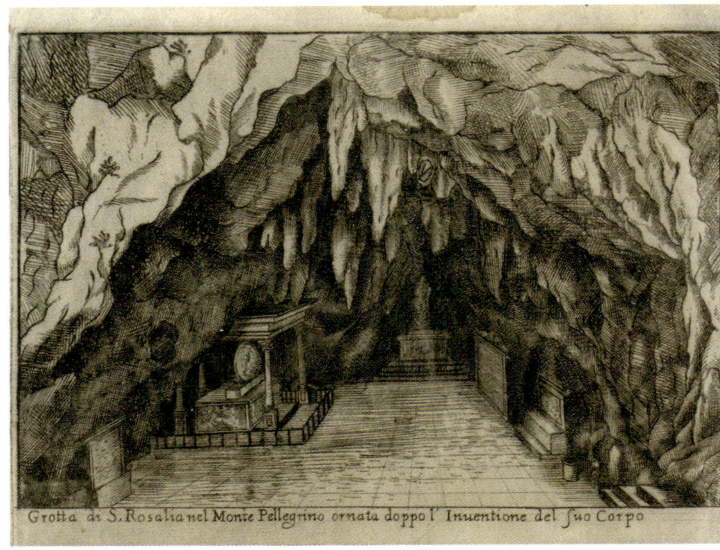
Grotta di S. Rosalia nel Monte Pellegrino ornata doppo l' Inuentione del ſuo Corpo

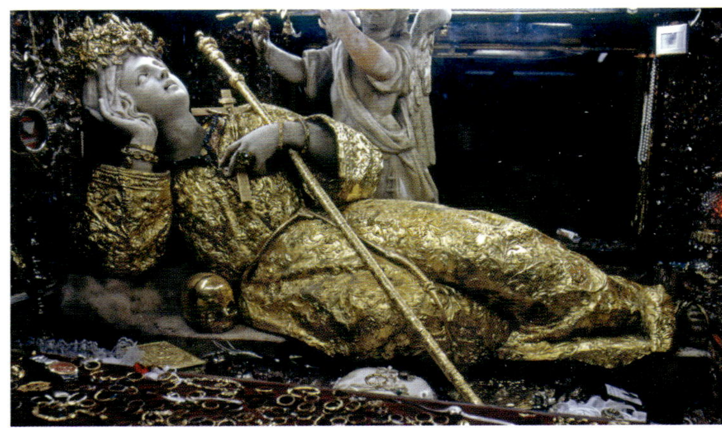

patrons were the members of the Compagnia del Rosario, whose oratory was attached to the church of San Domenico (fig. 31). On 22 August 1625, only a few weeks before leaving Palermo, Van Dyck signed a contract in the presence of the Governor, Francesco Barrale, and members of the Compagnia.[155] Pietro Martinelli, Giovan Giacomo Calderaio, and Antonio della Torre – a haberdasher from Genoa – were the three members named in the contract. The painter, tellingly, agreed to paint the altarpiece for the Compagnia 'in the city of Naples or in another place in Italy', showing that he had already planned to leave Palermo by that date.[156] It was specified that the large altarpiece should measure 15 by 10 ¾ *palmi* (the altarpiece is 397 × 278 cm) and that it should represent the Madonna of the Rosary with Saints Dominic, Vincent, Catherine of Siena, Rosalia, Christina, Ninfa, Oliva and Agatha. Van Dyck was to provide three coloured sketches 'and to send these to Palermo, or to deliver them in Naples, or in any other location, to an agent of the said Barrales or of the said della Torre'.[157] The three coloured *modelli* provided to the Compagnia do not survive, but two drawings for the altarpiece exist, a full sketch in a private collection (fig. 32), and a study for the head of Christ, in the Uffizi.[158] The contract specified that Van Dyck was to 'start, continue and finish the said painting well, diligently and skilfully, with fine pigments and of good quality, and in particular the blue colour for the Virgin's robes and other things of the said painting should be fine ultramarine'.[159] The altarpiece was to be delivered within February 1626, and once it had been finished it was to have been examined by two experts to determine that it had been painted to the satisfaction of the Compagnia. It was agreed that Van Dyck was to be paid 260 Neapolitan ducats for the painting.

The altarpiece was to replace another painting by Caravaggio's friend and follower Mario Minniti, who had been paid 100 *onze* on 19 December 1621 by Marco Gezio '*sacrae Teologie Doctor Magister Cappellanus Catedralis Ecclesie*'.[160] Minniti's altarpiece, 12 *palmi* high, was considered unsatisfactory and a new painting was commissioned from Van Dyck only four years later. It is likely that the Compagnia, after the plague of 1625, felt the need to have a new canvas that included the figure of Saint Rosalia, but it is also possible that by the mid-1620s Minniti's strictly Caravaggesque style was considered old-fashioned and the patrons preferred Van Dyck's neo-Venetian, and more modern manner.[161] Minniti's altarpiece entered Gezio's own private collection.

Van Dyck's *Madonna of the Rosary* was largely painted in Genoa, and the artist did not complete it within the six months established by the contract. The altarpiece finally reached Palermo on 8 April 1628, when Antonio della Torre was paid for his expenses in organising the transportation of the painting to Sicily.[162] Years later, on 1 April 1641 – eight months before Van Dyck died in London – della Torre and his brother-in-law Bartolomeo Rossetti, wrote to Cornelis de Wael in Genoa that 'I would be grateful to have some news of signor Anthony van Dyck', demonstrating that almost twenty years after the altarpiece was commissioned, one of the members of the Compagnia still remembered Van Dyck fondly.[163]

The altarpiece that Van Dyck painted for the Oratorio del SS. Rosario at San Domenico (fig. 33) is a magnificent and grandiose composition.[164] It has recently been portrayed as 'the first, and arguably the finest, great altarpiece of Van Dyck's oeuvre'.[165] Bellori described it in detail: 'he represented the Virgin in a glory of angels holding crowns, and below, Saint Dominic with the five Virgin Saints of Palermo, among them Saint Catherine and Saint Rosalia, with a putto nearby who puts his hand to his nose because of the stench of a dead man's head on the ground, a sign of the plague from which the city had been delivered through the intercession of the saints'.[166] Part of the composition was based on the altarpiece of the *Madonna of the Rosary* by Vincenzo da Pavia, dated 1540, in the left transept of San Domenico in Palermo, next to the oratory.[167] Van Dyck displayed in his altarpiece his understanding of sixteenth-century Venetian painting, in particular the religious works of Titian and Paolo Veronese; but he also paid a direct homage to his master, Rubens, in particular works like the *Madonna della Vallicella Worshipped by Saints* (Musée de Grenoble). The altarpiece is divided, as was a common tradition in Italy, between a divine sphere above and an earthly one, with saints, below. Against an architectural background of an arch framed by a pair of columns, the Virgin and Child appear on clouds. On each side are angels; some hold flowers (roses and lilies), one crowns the Virgin with roses, another holds a small flaming vase, while two present the Virgin with rosary beads. Mary offers a rosary to Saint Dominic, below her, who raises his right hand to accept it. To the left of Saint Dominic is Saint Vincent, and to the right of the arch, standing in her habit and crown of thorns, is Saint Catherine of Siena. The three Dominican saints – the Oratorio del SS. Rosario was attached to the main Dominican church of Palermo, San Domenico – are accompanied, as stipulated in the contract, by the five female saints of Palermo: Rosalia, Ninfa, Christina, Agatha and Oliva. Two of them are easily identifiable: Oliva is standing on the right, next to Catherine, holding a branch of olive. Rosalia is the kneeling saint, second from the left, in the brown habit and long flowing hair, who looks up to the Virgin and with her right hand points to the skull on the ground, replicating her iconography as protector against the plague in other paintings by Van Dyck. The three other female saints are more difficult to recognise, for the lack of specific attributes. The boy in the centre foreground, holding his nose, and fleeing from the pictorial into the spectator's space, is, as noticed by Bellori, a reference to the plague that hit Palermo in 1624, together with the overturned skull on the ground. A further plague saint, not mentioned in the original contract and not present in the preliminary sketch by Van Dyck, is Saint Sebastian, who is squeezed in at the extreme right, holding an arrow in his right hand.

By the time this splendid altarpiece reached Palermo, in 1628, Van Dyck had not been in the city for almost two years. Paradoxically, even though the canvas was painted entirely outside Palermo, this is the only work by the artist that survives to this day in the city. The oratory for which it was painted was drastically refashioned in the early eighteenth century, when the spectacular stuccowork by Giacomo Serpotta was commissioned, but Van Dyck's altarpiece still presides over the space, *in situ* in the oratory for which it was originally intended.

Epilogue

It has generally been assumed until recently that Van Dyck managed to leave Palermo as the plague struck the city, in the summer of 1624. The painter's stay in Sicily would have lasted, therefore, only a few months. Because of the lack of documents between July 1624 and August 1625 it was suggested that Van Dyck travelled around Italy in that period using Genoa as his principal home.[168] It was even rumoured that in July 1625 the painter travelled to Marseilles, but this is unlikely.[169] The discovery of a substantial group of documents in recent

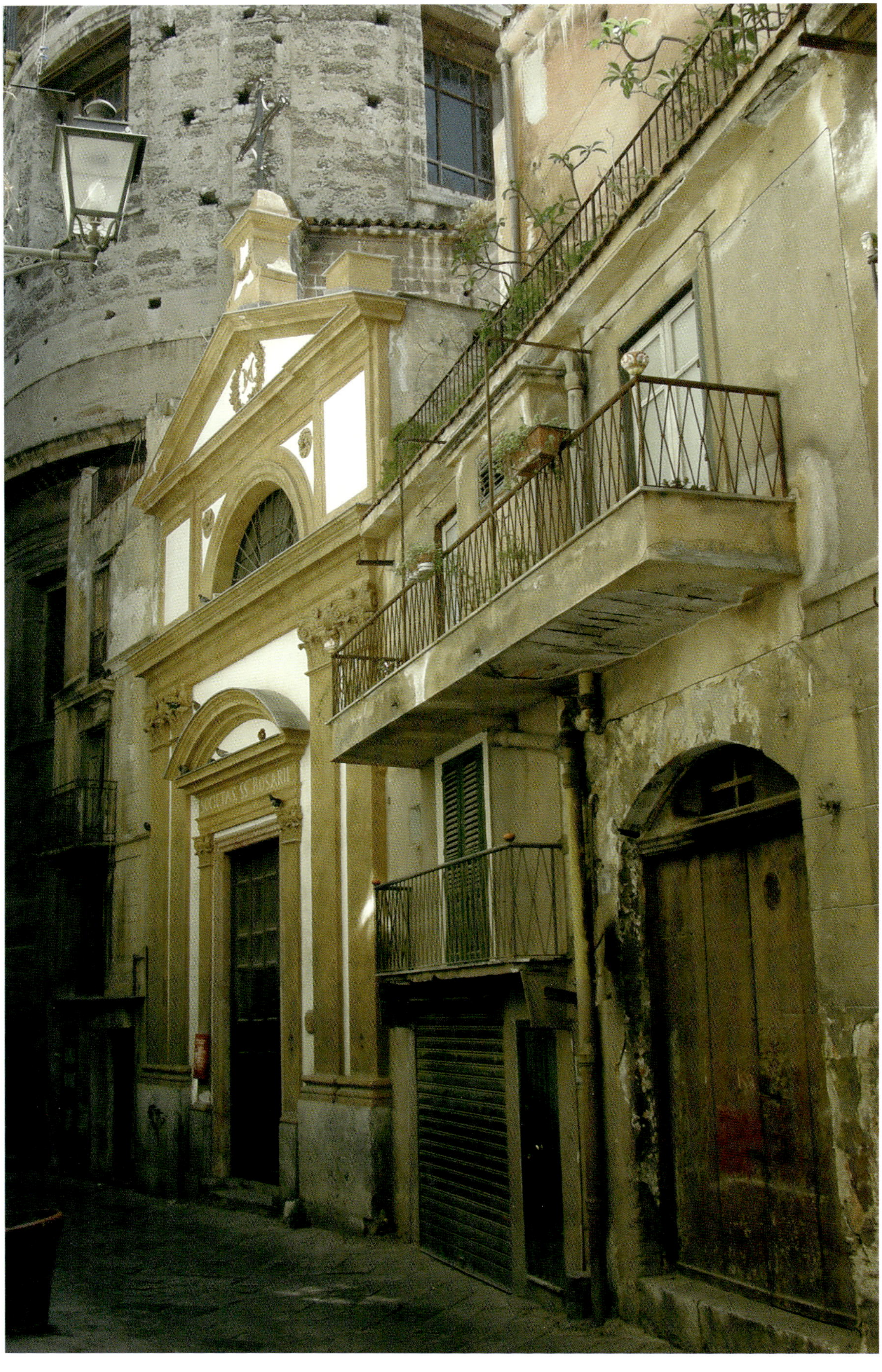

31 | Oratorio del SS. Rosario at San Domenico, Palermo

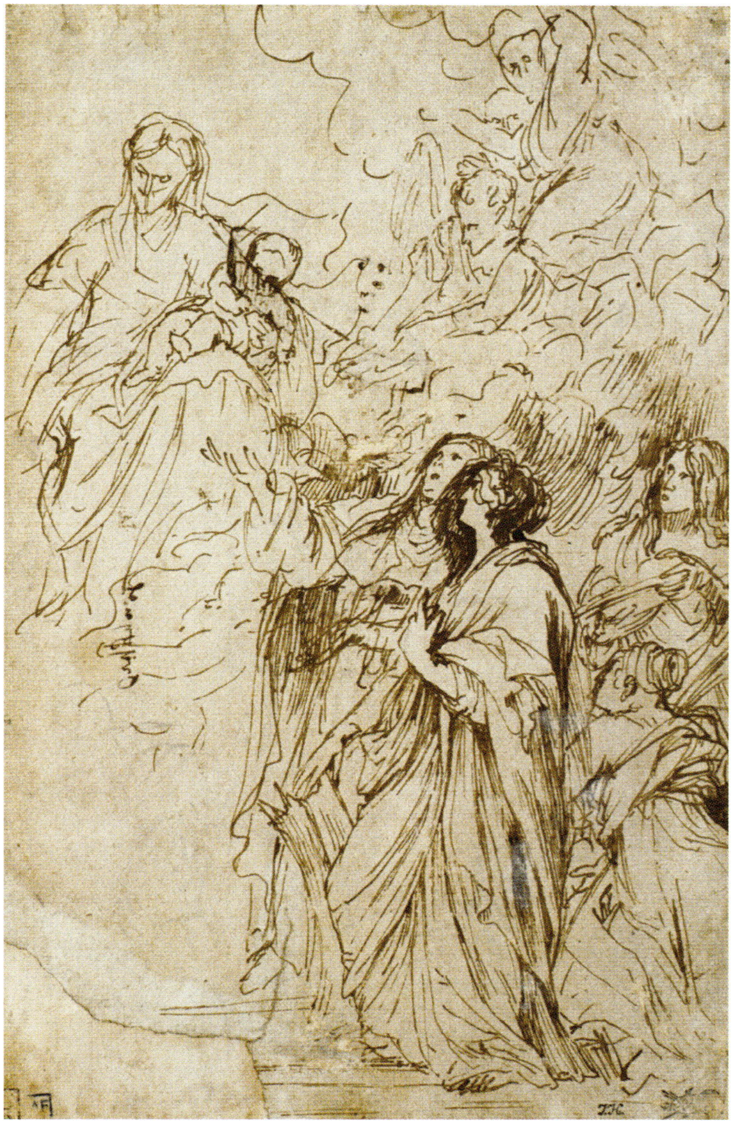

32 | Sir Anthony van Dyck,
Study for the Madonna of the Rosary
Private Collection

years has made it possible to understand that Van Dyck's sojourn in Sicily was actually much longer than it was envisaged before and that, at least until September 1625, the artist was based in Palermo.[170]

In his *Abecedario*, Pierre-Jean Mariette reported that the Genoese painter Bordone had given him an account of Van Dyck's escape from Palermo during the plague.[171] According to this adventurous version, the painter fled to Naples without the necessary bulletin of health; he was therefore arrested and condemned to the galleys.[172] Having given some of his drawings to the viceroy he was pardoned; and after a period working in Naples he returned to Genoa. Mariette's story can be discounted fairly easily as a romanticised version of the events surrounding Van Dyck's departure from Palermo. He may be correct, however, in reporting that when in the autumn of 1625 the artist left Sicily, he travelled to Naples. The contract for the altarpiece for the *Madonna of the Rosary* of August 1625 strongly suggests that Van Dyck was planning to travel to Naples and work on the altarpiece there. Two of the main foreign patrons in Naples, Ferdinand van den Eynden and Gaspar Roomer were from Antwerp. Van den Eynden had married Suzanne de Jode, whose sisters were the mothers of three of Van Dyck's close friends: Gertrude of Cornelis and Lucas de Wael, Isabelle of Jan Brueghel the Younger; and Roomer later owned two paintings by Van Dyck.[173] It seems reasonable that after September 1625, once the plague had been kept significantly under control, Van Dyck left Palermo and headed first to Naples and then returned to Genoa.

During his second Genoese sojourn, Van Dyck continued to create portraits and religious paintings for the local aristocracy, dealing with the network of Flemish and Genoese friends he had left behind when he travelled to Palermo in 1624. The period he had spent in Sicily, however, left a mark on him and many of his subsequent pictures are indebted to what he had produced in Palermo in 1624–25. The grandest portrait Van Dyck painted during his entire Italian career is that of the Lomellini family (fig. 34).[174] Relatives of Sofonisba Anguissola's husband, the five people in Van Dyck's painting are the family of Doge Giacomo Lomellini: his two eldest sons Nicolò and Giovan Francesco, his second wife Barbara Spinola and their two children Agostino and Vittoria. The large canvas was painted, around 1626, as war raged between Genoa and the Duke of Savoy (Emanuele Filiberto's father). The composition of the picture is a combination of motifs that Van Dyck had developed in his Italian years. The sitters – men, woman and children – are part of a visual language developed in some of the painter's greatest single portraits, such as *Cardinal Guido Bentivoglio* (fig. 3), *Elena Grimaldi Cattaneo* (fig. 4) or the *Portrait of a Boy* (fig. 5). The figure of Nicolò Lomellini, in particular, is based on that of Emanuele Filiberto in his portrait (cat. 2). The pose of Lomellini is similar to that of the viceroy, in reverse, and even in this case Van Dyck pays particular attention to the tour-de-force depiction of his sitter's armour. Very few of the men portrayed by Van Dyck in Italy were represented with armours. In this case, Nicolò's armour and the broken lance he

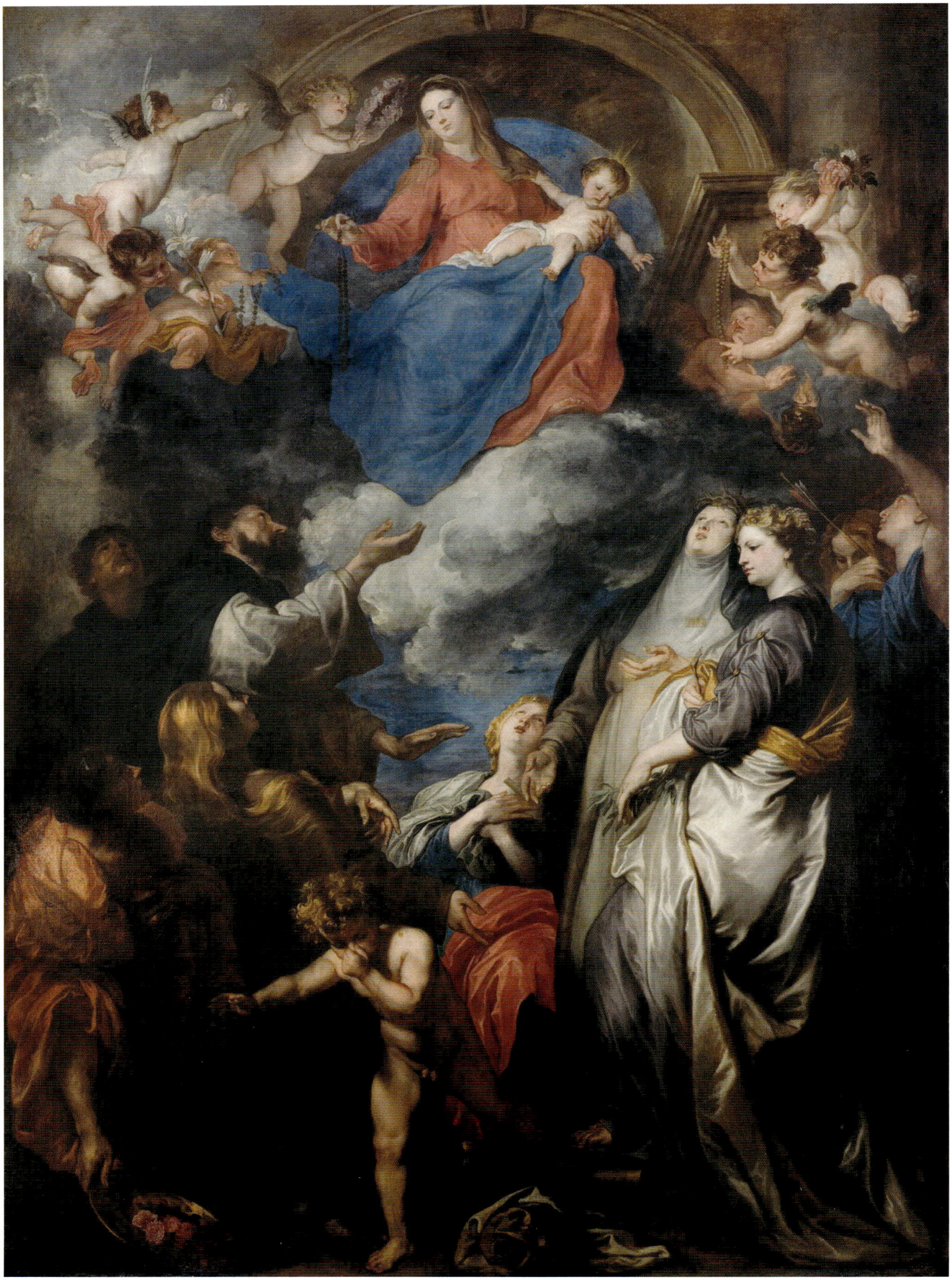

33 | Sir Anthony van Dyck
Madonna of the Rosary
Oratorio del SS. Rosario
at San Domenico, Palermo

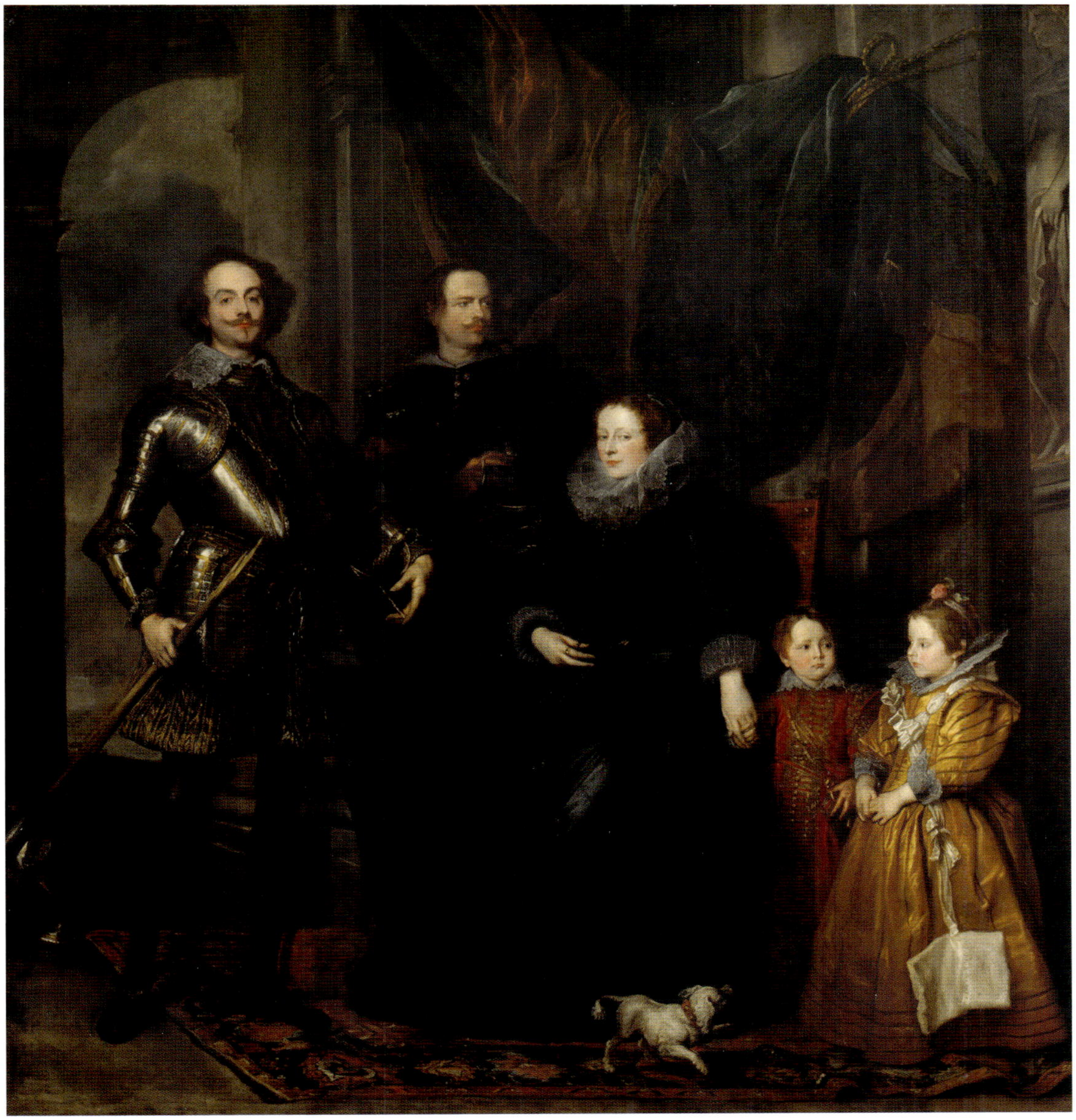

34 | Sir Anthony van Dyck,
The Lomellini Family
Scottish National Gallery, Edinburgh

clinches in his right hand are not signs of a dynastic upbringing but refer specifically to Lomellini's fighting in the war against the Duke of Savoy.

In May 1628 Van Dyck became a member of the Confraternity of Bachelors ('*Sodaliteit der bejaerde Jongmans*') in Antwerp; a few months later, in August, the same confraternity – closely linked to the Jesuits – acquired some relics of Saint Rosalia from Sicily. They were solemnly displayed in a chapel in the Jesuit church on 3 August 1628.[175] The Jesuits had been particularly keen to promote the cult of Rosalia in Europe, especially in France and in Flanders, and it was through their intervention that Pope Urban VIII included the saint in the *Martyrologium Romanum* in 1630. In 1629, Van Dyck painted an altarpiece for the confraternity's chapel; in it he depicted Saint Rosalia once again, reinterpreting in the composition of the work the lesson of Renaissance Venetian art (fig. 35).[176] A Titianesque Virgin is enthroned between the monumental figures of the apostles Peter and Paul; behind her colossal columns disappear behind clouds in the sky. The Child sits on the Virgin's lap and offers a crown of roses to the newly imported Sicilian saint, who kneels in front of them. While Rosalia's attributes – the skull, books and lilies – are placed, as a still life, on the steps of the throne, she appears dressed in unusually rich garments. For the Flemish confraternity, the simple, brown monastic robes worn by the hermit saint at the time of the plague gave way to a triumphal crimson outfit draped in a gold brocaded fabric. The painting is almost Van Dyck's *ex-voto* to Rosalia. As Charles Sterling commented in 1939, the painter must have felt 'a personal devotion, a faith, a profound gratitude to the saint for saving him', and the altarpiece was 'the last work of Van Dyck's representing St. Rosalie, the last echo of that terrible time when the thought of the Virgin of Palermo filled the artist's mind'.[177] While painting the confraternity's altarpiece, Van Dyck also worked on another project to do with the saint, providing the illustrations

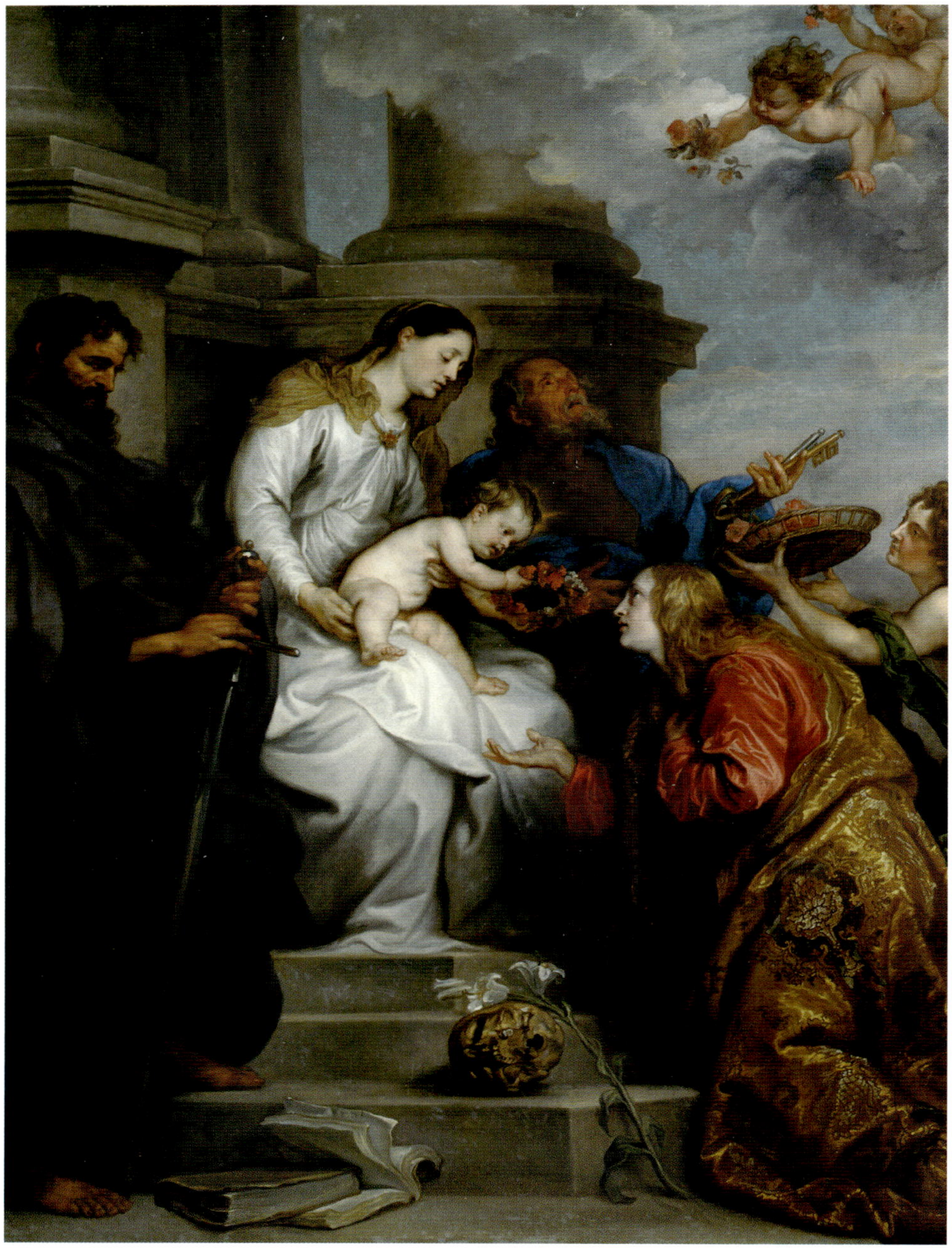

35 | Sir Anthony van Dyck,
The Virgin and Child with Saints Peter, Paul and Rosalia
Kunsthistorisches Museum, Vienna

for a small book on the life of Rosalia. The *Vita S. Rosaliae Virginis Panormitanae Pestis Patronae iconibus expressa*, published in Antwerp in 1629 by Cornelis Galle, included a series of images, engraved by Philip de Mallery that followed designs provided by Van Dyck, depicting events from the life of Saint Rosalia.[178] This is the only known example of the artist working on book illustrations, during his entire career.

Four years after leaving Palermo, Van Dyck returned to images of Saint Rosalia in Antwerp with his altarpiece and with the illustrations for the *Vita S. Rosaliae*. The year and a half spent in Sicily, among the unspeakable horrors of the plague, must have left a personal mark on him. Even in the midst of the pestilence, he continued to be active and painted at least two spectacular portraits (cats. 2 and 8), and large religious paintings (cats. 9 and 10). For a young artist the Sicilian capital must have been stimulating, and Van Dyck was visibly moved by his meeting with Sofonisba Anguissola (cat. 5) and documented with great interest what he saw in the streets in his sketchbook, from *commedia dell'arte* figures to the woman condemned as a witch. Notwithstanding the dangers caused by the plague, he was lucky to be in the city when the timely discovery of the bones of Saint Rosalia occurred. He quickly took over as the main painter of images of Rosalia, establishing her image on the island well into the future. This Sicilian experience left a mark on Van Dyck as a man and as an artist, and more importantly he himself, through his works, left a significant mark on Palermo and the artistic heritage of the island.

Notes

[1] 'Era egli ancor giovine, spuntando di poco la barba, ma la giovinezza sua veniva accompagnata da grave modestia di animo e da nobiltà di aspetto, ancorché picciolo di persona. Erano le sue maniere signorili più tosto che di uomo privato, e risplendeva in ricco portamento di abiti e divise, perché assuefatto nella scuola del Rubens con uomini nobili, ed essendo egli per natura elevato e desideroso di farsi illustre, perciò oltre li drappi si adornava il capo con penne e cintigli, portava collane d'oro attraversate al petto, con seguito di servitori,' Bellori 2009, p. 274; translated in Bellori 2005, p. 216.

[2] For Van Dyck's Italian period see Vaes 1924; Barnes 1986; Genoa 1997; S.J. Barnes in Barnes, De Poorter, Millar, Vey 2004, pp. 143–235; and Milan 2004.

[3] Larsen 1980a, pp. 118–19, cat. 462; P. Boccardo and C. Di Fabio in Genoa 1997, pp. 310–13, cat. 63; C. Brown in London 1999a, pp. 194–95, cat. 45; S.J. Barnes in Barnes, De Poorter, Millar, Vey 2004, pp. 210–11, cat. II.71.

[4] 'Tanto generoso che la sua casa era sempre aperta a tutti e massime a suoi nationali', Soprani 1674, p. 327.

[5] Larsen 1980a, p. 114, cat. 406; S.J. Barnes in Barnes, De Poorter, Millar, Vey 2004, pp. 175–76, cat. II.31.

[6] 'Et il n'a rien fait depuis qui le surpassat. Tout Rome accourut voir cette merveille de l'art, un chacun voulut être de la main de notre artiste,' Genoa 1997, p. 392; for the full text of the biography see Genoa 1997, pp. 391–92.

[7] Larsen 1980a, p. 115, cat. 411; S.J. Barnes in Genoa 1997, pp. 248–51, cat. 43; S.J. Barnes in Barnes, De Poorter, Millar, Vey 2004, pp. 189–90, cat. II.45.

[8] Larsen 1980a, p. 116, cat. 428; S.J. Barnes in Barnes, De Poorter, Millar, Vey 2004, pp. 216–17, cat. II.81.

[9] 'Venne desiderio ad Antonio di trasferirsi in Sicilia, dove trovandosi il principe Filiberto di Savoia allora viceré, fece il suo ritratto', Bellori 2009, p. 275; translated in Bellori 2005, p. 217.

[10] 'Emmanuel Philibert de Savoie, vice roi de cette île, et Grand-Prieur de Castille l'appella à sa cour en 1624 et lui fit un accueil très distingué', Genoa 1997, p. 392.

[11] Abbate 2004, p. 69.

[12] Vaes 1924, p. 216; Mendola 1999c, p. 60; Abbate 2004, p. 69.

[13] For more on Palermo in the seventeenth century, see Abbate 1999a; Palermo 1990a; Palermo 1999; Renda 2003; Servizi 2008.

[14] For art collecting in Palermo, see Abbate 1999b and Abbate 2011.

[15] Jaffé 2002, pp. 104–05, cat. 1067 (fol. 59) and 1068 (fol. 60). Jaffé 2002 and Brown 1982, pp. 84–85, identify the location of these scenes as Palermo. For Cust 1902, plate XX, they were drawn in Rome.

[16] 'Una striga in Palermo', Jaffé 2002, p. 104, cat. 1066 (fol. 58v). For a full discussion of the drawing see McGrath 2001.

[17] For witches, the Inquisition and trials in Sicily and more generally in Europe, see Bethencourt 1992; Briggs 1996; Messana 2007.

[18] McGrath 2001, p. 49.

[19] Mendola 1999b, p. 88; Mendola 1999c, p. 58; Abbate 2004, p. 69.

[20] Mendola 1999b, p. 88; Mendola 1999c, p. 58.

[21] Mendola 1999c, p. 63 n. 1; Abbate 2004, p. 69.

[22] Mendola 1999b, p. 88; Abbate 2004, p. 69.

[23] Abbate 1999a, pp. 38–43; Mendola 1999c, p. 60.

[24] For the church of San Giorgio dei Genovesi, see Patricolo 2006.

[25] Abbate 1999a, p. 56.

[26] Archivio di Stato, Palermo (hence ASP), Not. Francesco Sergio, stanza I, vol. 17619, ff. 306r–308r; also Not. Francesco Sergio, stanza I, vol. 17582, ff. 146r–148v; transcribed in Mendola 1999b, p. 97; Mendola 1999c, p. 60; Abbate 2004, p. 73.

[27] Susinno 1960, p. 166; Abbate 2004, p. 73.

[28] 'Quali ritratti il marchese di Pintidattilo, genero del predetto Ettore Vanactoven, ultimamente li regalò al marchese del Carpio, allorché venne da Roma al governo del regno di Napoli', Susinno 1960, p. 166; Abbate 2004, p. 73.

[29] ASP, Not. Francesco Sergio, stanza I, vol. 17619, ff. 771r–773r; Mendola 1999b, p. 97; Mendola 1999c, p. 60.

[30] ASP, Not. Francesco Sergio, stanza I, vol. 17619, f. 773r–774r ; Mendola 1999b, p. 99; Mendola 1999c, p. 60.

[31] Abbate 2004, pp. 73–74.

[32] ASP, Not. Francesco Sergio, stanza I, vol. 17619, ff. 873v–874r; Mendola 1999b, p. 99; Mendola 1999c, p. 60; Abbate 2004, p. 77.

[33] ASP, Not. Francesco Manso II, vol. 8098, f. 371v; vol. 8114, f. 246; Mendola 1999b, p. 99; Mendola 1999c, p. 60.

[34] ASP, Not. Matteo D'Alessandro, stanza II, vol. 3427, ff. 14r–14v; Mendola 1999c, p. 61 (who gives the wrong date of 3 December); Mendola 1999b, p. 99; Abbate 2004, p. 79.

[35] For Emanuele Filiberto of Savoy, see Litta 1872, plate XVI; Failla 2003.

[36] For the Ospedale see Failla 2003, pp. 16 n. 6, 40.

[37] For the inventories of Emanuele Filiberto, see Failla 2003.

[38] Failla 2003, pp. 40, 47–50.

[39] 'A Principis quadam effigie in terram labente judicium atque mens variorum. His dum intendit sui ad vivum effigiem delineari successivis horis patitur in Cubiculo Mosaico, ubi solus aliquando ratiocinatur, ubi sola est mensa, solum subsellium scribendo, et quiescendo commode perferte absoluta pictura superponitur mensae, cui multis insidet diebus. Princeps solus cubiculo claudit et aperit. Rediens a Missa sacris effigiem in faciem solo prostratam jacentem videt, nullo tunc manifesto flante vento, qui impetum fecerit, (numquam fere Panormi desunt venti). Picturae inter duas fenestras Palatii plateam respicientes positae ubi paries ventis, licet impetuose flantibus, resistere videtur. Sciscibatur num sciant, ut ceciderit effigies, nullo modo, aiunt Equites, quod nullus eo ingrediatur; male de salute, illiusque vita animantur ob picturae, nullo impellente, casum, quod mihi retulit Don Franciscus Manuel primus illius Aeconomus,' Matranga 1908, p. 13 n. 2, quoting a note in the copy of the *Vita Ser.mi Principis Filiberti a Sabaudo. Authore Ioanne Francisco Fiochetto Protomedico Ser.mi Sabaudiae Ducis, etc., anno Sal. M.D.C.XXVIII* in the Biblioteca Comunale in Palermo, f. 271. The original of the manuscript is in the Biblioteca Nazionale in Turin.

[40] Failla 2003, pp. 40–45.

[41] 'Fu nelle scienze morali e politiche, nelle naturali anche profondissimo, nelle matematiche poscia, nelle quali è stata tanta l'inopia degli Huomini buoni, che quasi appena uno per ogni secolo felice ne riesce, là dove nelle altre scienze innumerabili ne provengono, Filiberto divenne sì eccellente che ancora nella Meccanica, di quella artatissimamente di mani propria operava [...] rendono anco testimonio le carte da navigare, e gli altri strumenti in-

finiti maravigliosamente da lui divisati e fatti, per fregiare più che con altro caduto ornamento le sue glorie', Failla 2003, p. 46.
[42] Failla 2003, pp. 50–51.
[43] Failla 2003, pp. 52–57.
[44] Maya (no date).
[45] Maya (no date), pp. 1–9. '1624: Nel mese di Giugno venne in Trapani un Vascello di Tunisi, allo quale per complacenza del Viceré non se li fece fare la quarantena, com'è solito, solo se li fece far pochi giorni, e poi se ne venne in Palermo, et lassao la peste in Trapani, e la portò in Palermo; e si incominciano à poco à poco à trovarsi persone con buboni et suaposi, e ne morivano hora due, e tre il giorno; e doppo ne morivano a trenta, quaranta, et 70 lo giorno. Si fecero però li Capicento dell'Isole, e si fecero Carrozzoni, e seggette per li Infermi, e li morti sio portarono a seppellire fuori della Città alle Perriere, sotto le falde di Monte Pellegrino, con gran compassione del popolo; one ogn'uno vivo si piangea per morto. Si fece per la Città la Processione uscendo il Santissimo Crocifisso della Chiesa Maggiore, e si portò alla Chiesa della Madonna della Catena delli Padri Teatini; dove stette due giorni, con altre processioni; e poi si riportò alla Chiesa Maggiore. Durò il detto male circa due anni; per lo quale la Città spese circa sette cento mila scudi', Auria (no date), f. 56r.
[46] Maya (no date), pp. 10–13.
[47] Maya (no date), pp. 16–17.
[48] Maya (no date), pp. 17–19.
[49] Auria (no date), f. 56r.
[50] The 'Bando et Ordinationi fatte per l'Illustri & molto Spetabili Signori Offitiali della Felice Città di Palermo conchiuse e terminate nella Deputatione della Sanità sopra il morbo contagioso che corre nella detta Città' of 1625 is included in the *Raccolta sulla peste* (no page numbers).
[51] 'In primis che niuno debba entrare in questa nostra Città di Palermo, venendo da qual si voglia Città, o Terra, senza bolittino vero, & legitimo, da parte non sospetta, ne dichiarata per infetta', *Raccolta sulla peste*.
[52] 'Pena di quattro tratti di corda, & di remigiare nelle Regie galere per anni sette, se fosse persona ignobile, o vero povera, & essendo femina, oltra li quattro tratti di corda, di andare a servire allo Hospidale della Cubba per mesi quattro', *Raccolta sulla peste*.
[53] 'Et essendo persona nobile, o vero ricca di pagare onze cento, & di stare condennata in un Castello ben visto a detti Signori officiali per anni sette', *Raccolta sulla peste*.
[54] 'Sua Altezza il quale stando bene si levò di letto et andò il giorno di domenica adi 28 di Luglio in cocchio in fino à Porta Felice, e retornando in Palazo si ammalò', Auria (no date), f. 67v.
[55] 'Dalla Madre Chiesa sino a Palazo portando in quella processione il Corpo et la cassa di Santa Christina... et un quatro di Santa Rosolea che era delli Padri del Collegio', Auria (no date), f. 67v.
[56] Failla 2003, p. 62.
[57] For the issues to do with the inheritance, see Failla 2003, pp. 37–38, referring to documents in Archivio di Stato, Turin, Testamenti di Principi, mazzo 4, n. 12, *Testamento del Principe Emanuele Filiberto di Savoia*.
[58] 'La robba tutta si conserva ancora in casa intatta con vigilanza esattissima usata dal Sr Card Doria ma non si sa dire come stieno gli inventari né per mano di chi', Failla 2003, p. 38.
[59] 'Pensiero risolutissimo di recarvisi perché V.A. sia informata di ogni accidente', Failla 2003, p. 38.
[60] 'Alli 24 sul tardi, nilla ripa dove sbarcass.o concorse genti in grandissimo numero parendo loro miracolo il vedere quello che nilla conditione di questi miserissimi tempi rari volti si vede, cioè che vengano persone in quella città dalla quale per fuggiri i suoi pericoli tanto volentieri si ni partissero', Failla 2003, p. 38.
[61] 'Doria insiste che noi pagassimo con li nostri danari li debiti e ci pigliassimo questi robbi, ma il valore della robba non si può sapere in maniera alcuna', Failla 2003, p. 38.
[62] For the *Relación del Ynbentario de Bienes que dejo el ser.mo Pr.e Filiberto* see Failla 2003, p. 38.
[63] Abbate 1990, p. 40; Failla 2003, p. 37.
[64] Failla 2003, pp. 52, 64.
[65] The present tomb of Emanuele Filiberto was designed in the nineteenth century. Andres Ximenez (1764) describes what the tomb must have looked like in the eighteenth century: 'Cuerpos reales que estan en el Panteon pequeño [...] tres órdenes de Nichos para los Ataudes[...] son en todos cinqüenta y uno, y tienen otras tantas Targetas doradas, en cuyos campos se pone el Título de los Reales Cuerpos que los van ocupando; y como siguiendo el color de los Mármoles y Jaspes, se guarnecen de lo dorado, forman muy agradable vista con su diversidad [...] En el tercer órden: [...] El del Príncipe de Onella Don Manuel Filiberto, Gran Prior de San Juan, hijo de los dichos Señores Duques de Saboya Don Manuel, y Doña Catalina. Nació en Turin á diez y siete de Abril de mil quinientos ochenta y ocho. Murió en Palermo á tres de Agosto de mil seiscientos veinte y quatro. Fue trahído á esta Real Casa en veinte y uno de Diciembre de mil seiscientos veinte y cinco', pp. 360–61, 364.
[66] Abbate 2004, p. 70.
[67] For Sofonisba in Sicily, see Sacchi 1994.
[68] Abbate 2004, p. 70; Patricolo 2006, p. 175.
[69] For the Italian text, see cat. 5.
[70] Larsen 1980a, p. 114, cat. 418; Abbate 2004, pp. 70–71; Abbate 2011, p. 87.
[71] Abbate 2004, p. 71.
[72] 'SOPHONISBAE VXORI AB ANGVISSOLAE / COMITIBVS DVCENTI ORIGINE[M] PARENTV[M] / NOBILITATE FORMA EXTRAORDINARIJSQVE / NATVRAE DOTIBVS IN ILLVSTRES MVNDI MVLIE / RES RELATAE AC IN EXPRIMENDIS HOMINVM / IMAGINIBVS ADEO INSIGNI VT PARE[M] AETATIS SVAE / NEMINE[M] HABVISSE SIT AESTIMATA HORATIVS / LOMELLINVS INGENTI AFFECTVS MAERORE DECVS / HOC EXTREMVM ET SI TANTAE MVLIERI EXIGVVM / MORTALIBVS VERO MAXIMV[M] DICAVIT 1632'. For Sofonisba's tomb in San Giorgio dei Genovesi, see Patricolo 2006, pp. 172–76.
[73] Abbate 2004, p. 74.
[74] For the chapel, see Patricolo 2006, pp. 117–28.
[75] 'IOANNI AVGVSTINO SIGNO AMABILISSIMO GENTIS PRAESIDIO / FORTVNA ET GRATIA FLORENTISSIMO PIETATIS CVLTORI INTEGERRIMO / CVI OB CANDIDISSIMOS MORES INGENII EXCELLENTIAM / GENVENSIS NATIO BIS FASCES DETVLIT CONSVLARES / VITA FVNCTO INGENTIS AMORIS ET LACRYMARVM EXIGVVM MONVMENTVM / CAMILLA DE SIGNO ET VIGINTIMILLIS UXOR MOESTISSIMA / ET DESIDERIVS FILIVS EHU QVONDAM SVO VIVENTI POSVIT / VIXIT ANNOS LIII OBIIT ANNO MDCXX'. Patricolo 2006, p. 117.
[76] Patricolo 2006, p. 118.

[77] Abbate 1999a, p. 39; Abbate 2004, p. 74; Patricolo 2006, p. 121.
[78] Abbate 2004, p. 75.
[79] Abbate 2004, p. 75.
[80] Segno wrote his will on 12 December 1630 and his death certificate was signed on 17 December. Abbate 1990, p. 55 n. 62; Patricolo 2006, p. 118.
[81] The *Inventario degli oggetti mobili, rinvenuti nella casa mortuaria di D. Desiderio Segnio, estratto dall'atto compilato dal Notaro Pietro Lombardo di Salaparuta, nel dì 24 dicembre 1630* is transcribed by Di Giovanni 1889 but no location for the original document is given. The inventory was presumably in the archive of the palace at Salaparuta and lost in the earthquake that destroyed the town in 1968. See Appendix 2 for a full transcription.
[82] 'Un ritratto del quondam sign. Desiderio, di mano di Antonio Vandich, con guarnizione negra', Di Giovanni 1889, p. 287; Appendix 2.
[83] 'Un quatro di S. Rosalia in gloria, di mano di Antonio Vandich, con guarnizione negra. Un quatro di esposizione in croce, di mano dello stesso, con guarnizione come sopra. Un quatro con una testa che badiglia, di mano dello stesso Vandich, con guarnizione nigra et dorata', Di Giovanni 1889, p. 288; Appendix 2.
[84] 'Un quatro di un bagno di Ninfe, sopra pietra, di mano del Cambiaso, con guarnizione negra. Un quatro del ritratto di Amilcare Anguisciola, di mano della Signora Domina Sofonisba sua figlia', Di Giovanni 1889, p. 288; Appendix 2.
[85] ASP, Not. Francesco Comito, stanza I, vol. 923, f. 507r; Mendola 1999c, p. 61; Abbate 2004, p. 76.
[86] 'Die XXII Aprilis VIII Ind.e 1626. Quia Desiderius segno tenet apud se ut [...] quattro quadri del testamento vecchio con sue cornici nigre di altezza di sei palmi in circa, e di larghezza di sette palmi in circa che dicono siano di mano del Titiano ubi depicta sunt, videlicet: la sommersione di faraone, la cascata de la manna, la scaturition dell'acqua e lo sacrificio del vitello, nec non un quatro del martirio di Santo Stefano quod dicunt che sia di mano di Antonio Vandich fiamengo di altezza di nove palmi incirca, e sette palmi incirca di larghezza'. ASP, Not. Francesco Comito, stanza I, vol. 923, f. 507r; Mendola 1999c, p. 61; Abbate 2004, p. 76.
[87] Mendola 1999c, p. 62, relates the *Stoning of Saint Stephen* to a copy of the painting at Tatton Park once in a collection in Palermo and now untraced.
[88] Jaffé 2002, p. 73, cat. 989.
[89] Abbate 2004, p. 76.
[90] 'Apparteneva alla razza di quegli avventurieri che un secolo dopo l'Italia prodigherà all'Europa: i Casanova, i Cagliostro', Sciascia 1994, p. 16. '...Tra le tinte fosche del contrabbandiere di diamanti, quasi un demoniaco conte di Cagliostro ante litteram, e quella dell'avventuriero-connoisseur e del merchant-amateur', Abbate 1990, p. 42.
[91] Costello 1950, p. 257.
[92] Mendola 1999b, pp. 89, 104 n. 33.
[93] Mendola 1999b, pp. 89, 104 n. 34.
[94] Costello 1950, p. 258; Sciascia 1994, p. 15.
[95] Costello 1950, p. 259.
[96] ASP, Not. Antonio Mariano D'Amelia, vol. 1249, f. 238; Mendola 1999b, p. 89; Mendola 1999c, pp. 58–60.
[97] Abbate 2004, p. 76; Abbate 2011, p. 105, reasonably suggests that Valguarnera had given Segno the Gerards copies instead of the Titian originals.
[98] 'Mi maraviglio che V.S. non mi habbia dato risposta toccante il soggietto e misure del quadro chio sono obligato di fargli de mia mano propria. Io mi ritrovo una adoracione delli magi di sette a otto pied. d'altezza di forma quasi quadrata che non è finita di tuto punto e potria servire sopra l'altare di qualque capella privata et ancora per adornar la cheminea di un salon grande. Perciò desidero saper di V.S. se ella agradirebbe un tal soggietto pregandola mi faccia sapere la sua inclinacione liberamente con sicurta e chio sono disposto per servirla conforme ad ogni suo gusto e secondo l'obligo chio tengo a V.S. alla quale mi raccomando... Scrivo questo a caso non sapendo s'ella si trovi a Napoli o a Palermo o in altra parte pur spero ch'ella havra buon ricapito sapendo che gentilhuomini pari suoi sono consciuti da per tutto', Costello 1950, p. 282; Sciascia 1994, p. 17.
[99] 'Il Sig.re Ant.o Van Dijck rispose subito alla sua cortese lettera [avertendo] che il quadro era a buoniss.mo termine, et dice che inviera lo subito come scrisse anche a V.S. et mi fece grandiss.ma instanza che la tirasse inanti la rissolut.ne di quel quadro nel ritratto del Titiano. Il Sig.re Pietro Paolo mi rispose 14 giorni doppo, et subito che mi capitorno le recapitai per Palermo conforme l'ord.ne lasciatomi', Costello 1950, p. 281.
[100] For the two most complete accounts of the Valguarnera trial, see Costello 1950 and Sciascia 1994. All relevant documents are in Archivio di Stato, Rome, R. Chirografo 1630–2, Archivio del Governatore, processo contro F. Valguarnera.
[101] Costello 1950, p. 256.
[102] 'È Licentiato In Jure, mathematicus, et s'intende anco bene In varie sorte de medecine, qua ha guarrito Il s.e Rubbens dalla podagra', Costello 1950, p. 270.
[103] Costello 1950, pp. 267–68.
[104] Costello 1950, p. 268.
[105] Costello 1950, p. 268.
[106] Costello 1950, pp. 238–39.
[107] Costello 1950, p. 239.
[108] Costello 1950, pp. 271–72; Rome 1994, pp. 229–30.
[109] Costello 1950, p. 272.
[110] Rome 1994, pp. 233–34.
[111] 'Die 2 Januarij 1632. Questa matina è morto quel D. Fabritio Valguarnera che si trovava priggione in Tor di nona per la Causa del furto delli Diamanti, dopo essere stato ammalato d. febre molti giorni', Costello 1950, p. 279.
[112] Costello 1950, p. 260.
[113] Collura 1977, p. 51; Bailey 2005, p. 119.
[114] Collura 1994, p. 9; Bailey 2005, pp. 119, 121.
[115] Bailey 2005, pp. 119–21.
[116] Bailey 2005, p. 120.
[117] Di Natale 1994, p. 16; Vitella 1994, p. 83; Bailey 2005, p. 120.
[118] Collura 1977, pp. 80, 82.
[119] Di Natale 1994, p. 16; Abbate 2004, p. 77; Bailey 2005, p. 120.
[120] Collura 1977, pp. 80, 82; Di Natale 1994, pp. 16–18; Palazzotto 2003, pp. 11–13. The original reliquary of Saint Rosalia was subsequently used for the relics of Saint Agatha and is now in the Cappella delle Reliquie in the Cathedral of Palermo. The present silver reliquary of Saint Rosalia was designed in 1631–37 by Mariano Smiriglio, and made by four silversmiths, Giuseppe Oliveri, Francesco Rivelo, Giancola Viviano and

Matteo Lo Castro, in collaboration with Michele Ferruggia and Francesco Roccuzzo; for this see Collura 1977, p. 85; Di Natale 1994, pp. 11–80.

[121] '1624: In detto anno si ritrovò il corpo della nostra Cittadina di Palermo Santa Rosalia, in una grotta del Monte Pellegrino, dove anticamente haveva habitato come romita. Il suo corpo fu portato al Cardinale Doria, Arcivescovo di Palermo, il quale doppo molte consulte di Teologi declarò essere il corpo di essa santa, stante l'antiche historie, e traditioni, e molti miracoli adoperati da detta Santa, la quale andava comparendo à diverse persone infette del morbo contagioso, sanandole dallo infetto, anzi diceva che comparissiro dove il detto Cardinale, e si dicessero che quello che haveva in suo potere era il suo corpo, e che non ci havesse più dubbio nessuno; aggiungendo che declarato che seria, e fatta la Processione haveria dell'intutto cessato il male del contaggio. Onde finalmente finite le dispute delli Teologi ed altre persone dotte, declarò il Cardinale quello essere il vero corpo di Santa Rosalia; e cosi nell'anno seguente 1625: si fece la Processione, e la Città fece uno Arco Trionfale, con tanta sollennittà, alle quattro cantonere, che passò la loro altezza. Si fecero anco altri Archi Trionfali da diverse nationi per tutte le strade dove passava la detta Processione; la quale doppo che si fece cessò la peste, per gratia di Dio et intercessione di detta Santa miracolosa', Auria (no date), f. 56r.

[122] '...Quantunque si debba sperare la liberatione del morbo contagioso per l'intercessione della gloriosa SANTA ROSALIA Patrona, e Cittadina di questa Città; non per questo si debbono lasciar da parte li mezzi e diligenze humane', see Appendix 1, doc. 2.

[123] See Appendix 1, doc. 1.

[124] See Appendix 1, doc. 3.

[125] See Appendix 1, doc. 3.

[126] Bailey 2005, p. 123.

[127] For the first *Festino* see Vitella 1994.

[128] For the iconography of Saint Rosalia see Collura 1977 and Bailey 2005.

[129] Collura 1977, p. 96; Bailey 2005, p. 124.

[130] Collura 1977, p. 96.

[131] Sterling 1939, p. 61.

[132] Bailey 2005, p. 125.

[133] Bailey 2005.

[134] Bailey 2005, pp. 118, 125–27.

[135] Bailey 2005, pp. 127–28.

[136] Sterling 1939, p. 54; Larsen 1980a, p. 118, cat. 453; Bailey 2005, pp. 128–29.

[137] For the copy in Palermo, see Mendola 1999b, p. 101; Mendola 1999c, p. 62. For the Ciminna altarpiece see Abbate 1991, pp. 100, 102.

[138] Bailey 2005, pp. 131–33.

[139] Bailey 2005, pp. 119, 131–33.

[140] Sterling 1939, p. 62.

[141] See Appendix 2.

[142] 'Lo ritratto di esso testatore quattro quatri fatti di mano di ant[oni]o vandic Fiamingo'. The will of Sitaiolo is in ASP, Not. Giovanni Lo Piccolo, stanza II, vol. 1481, ff. 191r–197r. For the mention of the Van Dyck portrait, see f. 196r. See also Mendola 1999b, p. 101; Mendola 1999c, p. 61; Abbate 2004, p. 74. It is unclear, however, if the portrait of Sitaiolo is, like the other four paintings, also by Van Dyck. The inventory of Sitaiolo's pictures (see below) does not specify that the portrait is by Van Dyck.

[143] 'Item un quatro di un Satiro di mano di ant vandic con suo panno de taffita russo et sua bacchetta di ferro, Item un quatro grande di San gio: di mano di ant vandic con taffita del proprio modo [...] Item un quatro di sancta rosolea di mano di vanic (sic!) con lo suo taffita carmixino et bachetta [...] Item un quatro della Madonna con no[st]ro Sig[no]re in bracza sancta rosolea et san Joanne di mano di vandic'. The inventory is in ASP, Not. Giovanni Lo Piccolo, stanza II, vol. 1481, ff. 222r–237v; for the section on paintings (ff. 234r–234v). See also Mendola 1999b, p. 101; Mendola 1999c, p. 61; Abbate 2004, p. 74.

[144] Mendola 1999b, p. 101.

[145] 'Item un quatro della Magdalena con sua cornici dorata e sua taffità torchina del Vandich [...] item un quatro di Santo Antonino con sua cornici dorata del Vandich [...] item un quatro della Madonna con suo puttino con sua corona in mano con sua cornici dorata e sua taffità allandrata del Pandich (sic!) [...] item un quatro di un Christo morto in bracza della Madonna con san Giovanne e la Magdalena con sua cornici dorata del Vandich [...] item un quatro della Madonna del Rosario con diversi figorini con sua cornici dorata del Vandich [...] item un quatro della Madonna con suo puttino in bracza con sua cornici dorata e nigra del Vandich', Morreale 1999, p. 145. See also Mendola 1999b, p. 101; Mendola 1999c, p. 61; Abbate 1990, p. 37; Abbate 2004, p. 77.

[146] 'Tela ad'oglio di santa Rosalia di palmi cinque e quattro con cornice di noce toccata d'oro di mano di Vandike', Morreale 1990, p. 44; See also Mendola 1999b, p. 101; Mendola 1999c, p. 61; Abbate 2004, p. 77.

[147] Morreale 1990, pp. 149–52; See also Mendola 1999b, p. 101; Mendola 1999c, p. 61; Abbate 2004, p. 77.

[148] 'Un quatro della Madonna col puttino del Vandich con sua cornice dorata a crocciola [...] un quatro di Nostra Signora della Pietà mano di Vandich', Abbate 1990, p. 29; see also Mendola 1999b, p. 101; Mendola 1999c, p. 61.

[149] 'È oz. 5 – per compra di tre teste Et uno Corpuzzo di Creta cotto del Michelangelo Bonaroti Et le teste una sopra carta testa di Satiro di Mano di Ant. Vandijch l'Altre due del Monrealese Et suo figlio dico oz. 5', Ruffo 1916, p. 31.

[150] 1 January 1652: 'E più dui quadri e una testa d'Antonio Vandichi fiamengho, cioè uno, di palmi 3 e 4 e mezzo, con una santa Rosolia et undici angioletti che la tirano in cielo, costò in Palermo onze 26, onze 3 di cornice, et onze 1 di nolo, in tutto onze 30; et onze 24 per uno ritratto d'un pittore, con tutta la cornice, di palmi 4 e 5; et onze 2 una testa d'un satiro sopra carta; in tutto sono onze 59. E sono li dui quadri grandi vincolati'; 1 January 1668: 'Antonio Mandic [sic], dui quadri, di palmi 5 e 4 in circa, uno d'un ritratto d'un dottore che tiene un libro in mano, altro di santa Rosolia accompagnata d'11 puttini'; 1677: 'Antonio Vandich, quadri dui, di palmi 4 e 5 in circa per ciascheduno, cioè uno di santa Rosolia accompagnata da 11 puttini che la tirano in cielo, figura di 4 palmi in circa; et un altro d'un dottore, d'una meza figura, ritratto d'un dottore scoperto che tiene un libro in mano, ambedue quadri con cornici intagliati et indorati'. De Gennaro 2003, pp. 69–70, 107, 126, nos. 322, 483, 587.

[151] 'Sbozzi di Vannic in carta ogliati', Abbate 1990, p. 50; Mendola 1999b, p. 101; Mendola 1999c, p. 61.

[152] 'Sancta Rosolea copiata d'Antonio Bandichi con la Gloria dell'angeli conforme a quillo copiato d'Antonio Bandichi', in ASP, Not. Vincenzo Lenza, vol. 2678, f. 966; Mendola 1999b, p. 101; Mendola 1999c, p. 61.

[153] 'In primis un'Annunziata non complita copia del Vandic di palmi 4 e 5 [...] un quatro con la Madonna S. Rosalia et altri figuri copia del Vandic di palmi 8 e 10', Abbate 1990, p. 50; Mendola 1999b, p. 101; Mendola 1999c, p. 61.
[154] ASP, Not. Salvatore Miraglia, vol. 424, f. 1970; Mendola 1999b, p. 101; Mendola 1999c, p. 61.
[155] For the contract see Appendix 3; see also Mendola 1999b, p. 99; Mendola 1999c, p. 60; Abbate 2004, p. 79.
[156] 'Depingere nella città di Napoli, o in altro luogo d'Italia', see Appendix 3.
[157] 'Sia tenuto fare tre disegni coloriti, e quelli inviare qua in Palermo, o consegnarli in Napoli, o in altro luogo al commissionaro di d[ett]o di Barrales, o di d[ett]o della torre', see Appendix 3.
[158] C. Brown in New York and Fort Worth 1991, pp. 167–68, cat. 45; Bolten and Folmer-von Oven 1989, p. 226, cat. 127.
[159] 'Sia tenuto cominciare, seguitare e finire il detto quatro bene, diligente, e magistrevolmente con colori fini e di buona conditione, et in particolare che il colore torchino per il manto della Madonna, et altre cose di d[ett]o quatro sia oltra marino fino', see Appendix 3.
[160] Abbate 2004, p. 80.
[161] Abbate 2004, p. 80; Abbate 2011, p. 98.
[162] Mendola 1999b, p. 99; Abbate 2004, p. 81.
[163] 'Ne sarò grato aver qualche nova del Sig. Antonio Vandijch', Vaes 1925, pp. 214–15; Abbate 1990, pp. 47, 50; Abbate 2004, p. 81.
[164] For the painting see Sterling 1939, p. 60; Larsen 1980a, p. 117, cat. 441; Barnes 1986, pp. 51–54, 154–58, cat. 8; S. Barnes in Barnes, De Poorter, Millar, Vey 2004, pp. 153–55, cat. II.7.
[165] S. Barnes in Barnes, De Poorter, Millar, Vey 2004, p. 153.
[166] 'Espresse la Vergine in Gloria di Angeli che tengono le corone, e sotto San Domenico con le cinque Sante Vergini palermitane, tra le quali Santa Caterina e Santa Rosaria, con un putto appresso che si pone la mano al naso per lo fetore d'una testa di morto in terra, contrasegno del morbo da cui la città si era liberata per l'intercessione de' Santi', Bellori 2009, p. 276; translated in Bellori 2005, p. 217.
[167] Barnes 1986, p. 52.
[168] Genoa 1997, p. 386.
[169] Mendola 1999c, p. 61.
[170] The key documents have been discovered and published by Giovanni Mendola. See Mendola 1999b; Mendola 1999c.
[171] Mariette 1851, vol. 2, p. 175.
[172] Vaes 1924, p. 217 n. 3.
[173] Abbate 2004, p. 81.
[174] For the portrait, see Cust 1900, p. 243, cat. 106; Glück 1931, p. 194; Larsen 1980a, pp. 115–16, cat. 419; Barnes 1986, pp. 337–40, cat. 84; Larsen 1988, p. 147, cat. 362; Genoa 1997, pp. 73–74, 278–81, cat. 53; C. Brown in London 1999a, pp. 186–87, cat. 41; S. Barnes in Barnes, De Poorter, Millar, Vey 2004, pp. 192–93, cat. II.49.
[175] Sterling 1939, p. 60.
[176] For the altarpiece, see Sterling 1939, pp. 60–61, Larsen 1980b, p. 98, cat. 646, H. Vey in Barnes, De Poorter, Millar, Vey 2004, p. 285, cat. III.50; Bailey 2005, p. 131.
[177] Sterling 1939, p. 60.
[178] For the illustrations and the book, see Filipczak 1989.

Catalogue

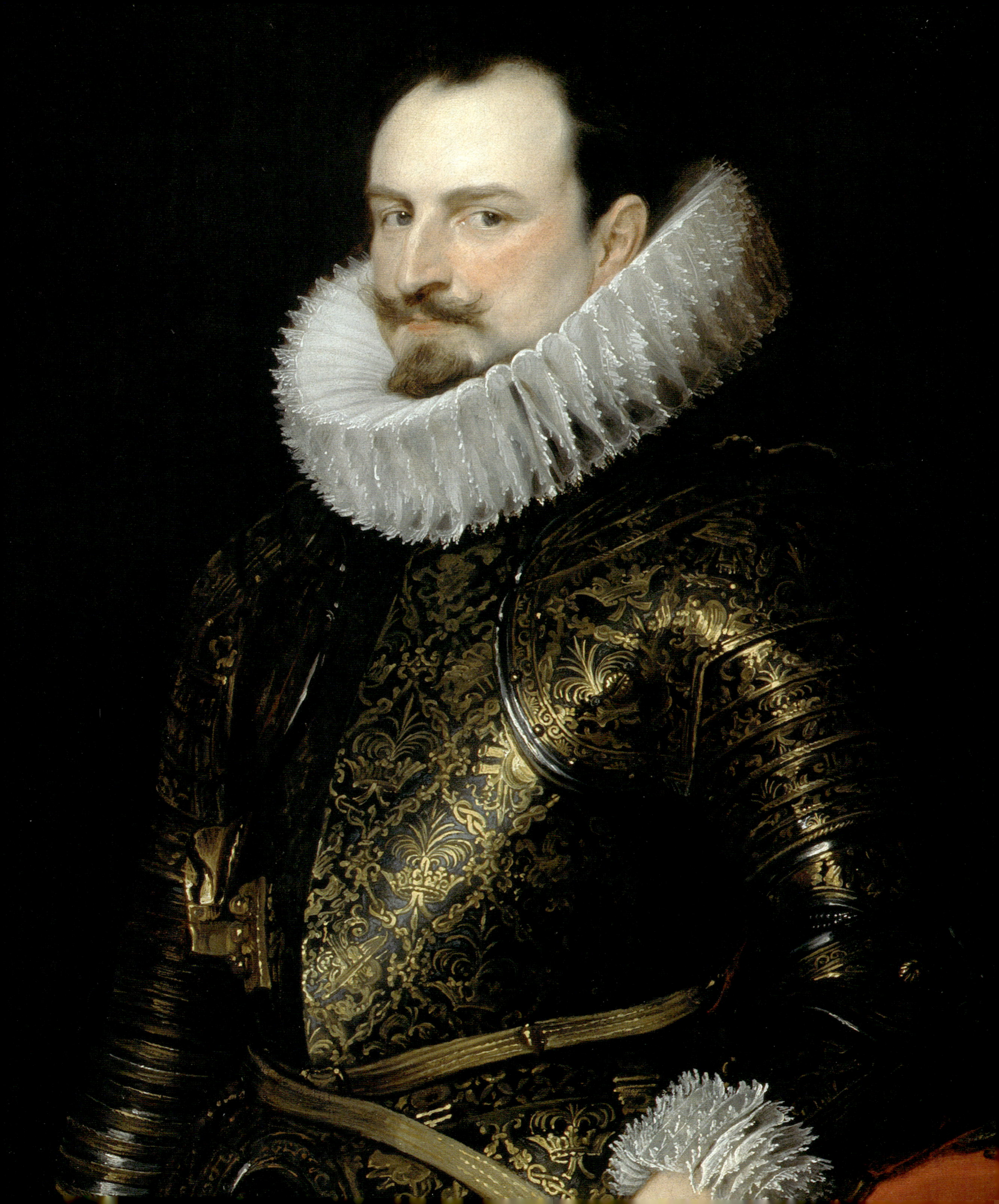

Van Dyck in Sicily:
the Viceroy Emanuele Filiberto of Savoy

1 | Sir Anthony van Dyck
(1599–1641)

Self-Portrait

c. 1620–21
Oil on canvas, 119.7 × 87.9 cm
The Metropolitan Museum of Art, New York
The Jules Bache Collection, 1949 (49.7.25)

PROVENANCE

Henry Bennet, 1st Earl of Arlington (1618–85), Euston Hall, near Thetford, Norfolk, by 1677; his daughter, Isabella, Duchess of Grafton (d. 1722/23); the Dukes of Grafton, Euston Hall; Alfred William Maitland Fitzroy, 8th Duke of Grafton (1850–1930); Christie's, London, 13 July 1923 (lot 143); Hopkins; Duveen Brothers, New York and Paris, 1924; Jules S. Bache (1861–1944), New York; gift of Jules Bache, 1949.

In his biography of Van Dyck, Giovan Pietro Bellori (2005, p. 216; 2009, p. 274) described the young artist in Rome in 1622: 'he was still young, his beard barely sprouting, yet his youth was accompanied by grave modesty of character and nobility of mien, albeit he was small in stature. His manners were those of a lord rather than a commoner, and he appeared resplendent in rich attire of suits and court dress' ('era egli ancor giovine, spuntando di poco la barba, ma la giovinezza sua veniva accompagnata da grave modestia di animo e da nobiltà di aspetto, ancorché picciolo di persona. Erano le sue maniere signorili più tosto che di uomo privato, e risplendeva in ricco portamento di abiti e divise'). The *Self-Portrait* in the Metropolitan Museum is one of the earliest by the artist, and depicts him as a stylish gentleman rather than as a painter. The canvas is first described by John Evelyn on the occasion of a dinner, on 16 November 1677, which he attended with his son, at the house of the Lord Chamberlain, Henry Bennet, 1st Earl of Arlington. Evelyn recalled 'two Vandyke's, of which one was his own picture at length, when young, in a leaning posture; the other an eunuch, singing. Rare pieces indeed!' Through Arlington's daughter, Isabella, the painting entered the collection of the Dukes of Grafton, and there it was recorded by Horace Walpole: 'at the Duke of Grafton's is a fine half length of Vandyck by himself, when young, holding up his arm, the hand declined'. It remained in the Grafton collection until sold at auction in 1923, and a year later it was acquired by Jules Bache in New York.

The painting is closely related to two other *Self-Portraits*, in the State Hermitage Museum in Saint Petersburg (fig. 1) and in the Alte Pinakothek in Munich (S.J. Barnes in Barnes, De Poorter, Millar, Vey 2004, pp. 138, 169–71, cats. I.59, II.26). The dating of the three paintings and their relative chronology has been the source of much speculation. Smith (1831, p. 211) originally proposed that the New York portrait dated from 'around the time he resided at Genoa', but Lionel Cust (1900, p. 211) already noticed that it was more likely painted 'before 1621'. The *Self-Portrait* is particularly close to Van Dyck's work from his first Antwerp period. However, the provenance suggests, as rightly proposed by Walter Liedtke (1984a), that the painting should date from the artist's first English sojourn, around 1620–21. The flesh tones and the hands in the *Self-Portrait* are particularly close in treatment to the ones in the *Continence of Scipio* (Christ Church Picture Gallery, Oxford) painted around 1620–21 in London, probably for the Duke of Buckingham (O. Millar in Barnes, De Poorter, Millar, Vey 2004, pp. 135–36, cat. I.57).

The *Self-Portrait* was painted over a re-used canvas, and the portrait of a man with a moustache and goatee is visible in X-ray photographs of the work, to the left of the artist's head (fig. 36). The twenty-one-year-old painter was already clearly influenced by Venetian portraiture – especially by Titian – in his refined technique, and in creating a supremely sophisticated image. The Munich *Self-Portrait* was originally closer in composition to the New York one, as X-rays revealed the same posture for the hand in its earlier version. It seems likely that both the Munich and Saint Petersburg paintings slightly post-date the New York one and were probably painted in Italy.

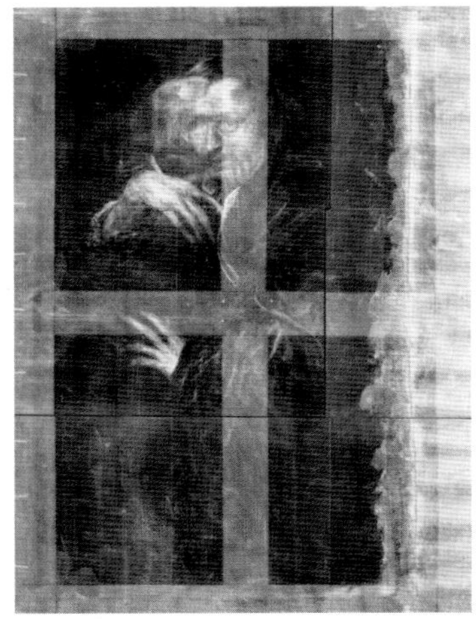

36 | Sir Anthony van Dyck, X-ray of *Self-Portrait*
The Metropolitan Museum of Art, New York

SELECT BIBLIOGRAPHY

Walpole 1828, vol. 2, p. 223; Smith 1831, vol. 3, pp. 210–11; Evelyn 1850, vol. 2, p. 109; Cust 1900, pp. 19, 203, 211, 221, 235; London 1900, p. 35, cat. 87; Brandus 1928, p. 194; Glück 1931, p. 532; Glück 1934, pp. 195–96; Van Puyvelde 1950, pp. 96, 125, 130, 172; Larsen 1980a, p. 103, cat. 254; A. McNairn in Ottawa 1980, pp. 8, 26, 165–66, cat. 76; Brown 1982, pp. 52–53; Liedtke 1984a, pp. 67–71; Liedtke 1984b, pp. 4, 18, 20; Larsen 1988, p. 28, cat. 41; Liedtke 1989, pp. 161–64; S.J. Barnes in Barnes, De Poorter, Millar, Vey 2004, p. 138, cat. I.60; C. Brown in London 1999a, p. 164; K. Hearn in London 2009, p. 47, cat. 5.

EXHIBITIONS

Exhibition of the Works of Sir Anthony van Dyck, Grosvenor Gallery, London 1887, cat. 93; *Van Dijk Tentoonstelling*, Koninklijk Museum voor Schone Kunsten, Antwerp 1899, cat. 54; *Exhibition of Works by Van Dyck*, Royal Academy of Arts, London 1900, cat. 87; *Loan Exhibition of Dutch Paintings of the Seventeenth Century*, Detroit Institute of Arts, Detroit 1925, cat. 30; *Eighth Loan Exhibition of Old Masters. Paintings by Anthony van Dyck*, Detroit Institute of Arts, Detroit 1929, cat. 12; *Masterpieces of Art: European Paintings and Sculpture from 1300–1800*, World's Fair, New York 1939, cat. 98; *The Bache Collection*, The Metropolitan Museum of Art, New York 1943, cat. 25; *Metropolitan Museum Masterpieces*, Hofstra College, Hempstead, New York 1952, cat. 4; *Picture of the Month*, Akron Art Institute, Akron 1952; *Portrait of the Artist*, The Metropolitan Museum of Art, New York 1972, cat. 7; *The Young Van Dyck*, National Gallery of Canada, Ottawa 1980, cat. 76; *Dutch and Flemish Painting in Norfolk*, Castle Museum, Norwich 1988, cat. 13; *From El Greco to Cézanne: Masterpieces of European Painting from the National Gallery of Art, Washington and The Metropolitan Museum of Art, New York*, National Gallery Alexandros Soutzos Museum, Athens 1992–93, cat. 8; *The Metropolitan Museum of Art, New York: Chefs-d'œuvre de la peinture européenne*, Fondation Pierre Gianadda, Martigny 2006, cat. 16; *Grandes maestros de la pintura europea de The Metropolitan Museum of Art, Nueva York: De El Greco a Cézanne*, Museu Nacional d'Art de Catalunya, Barcelona 2006–07, cat. 12; *Van Dyck & Britain*, Tate Britain, London 2009, cat. 5; *Rubens & Van Dyck*, Nationalmuseum, Stockholm 2010, cat. 30.

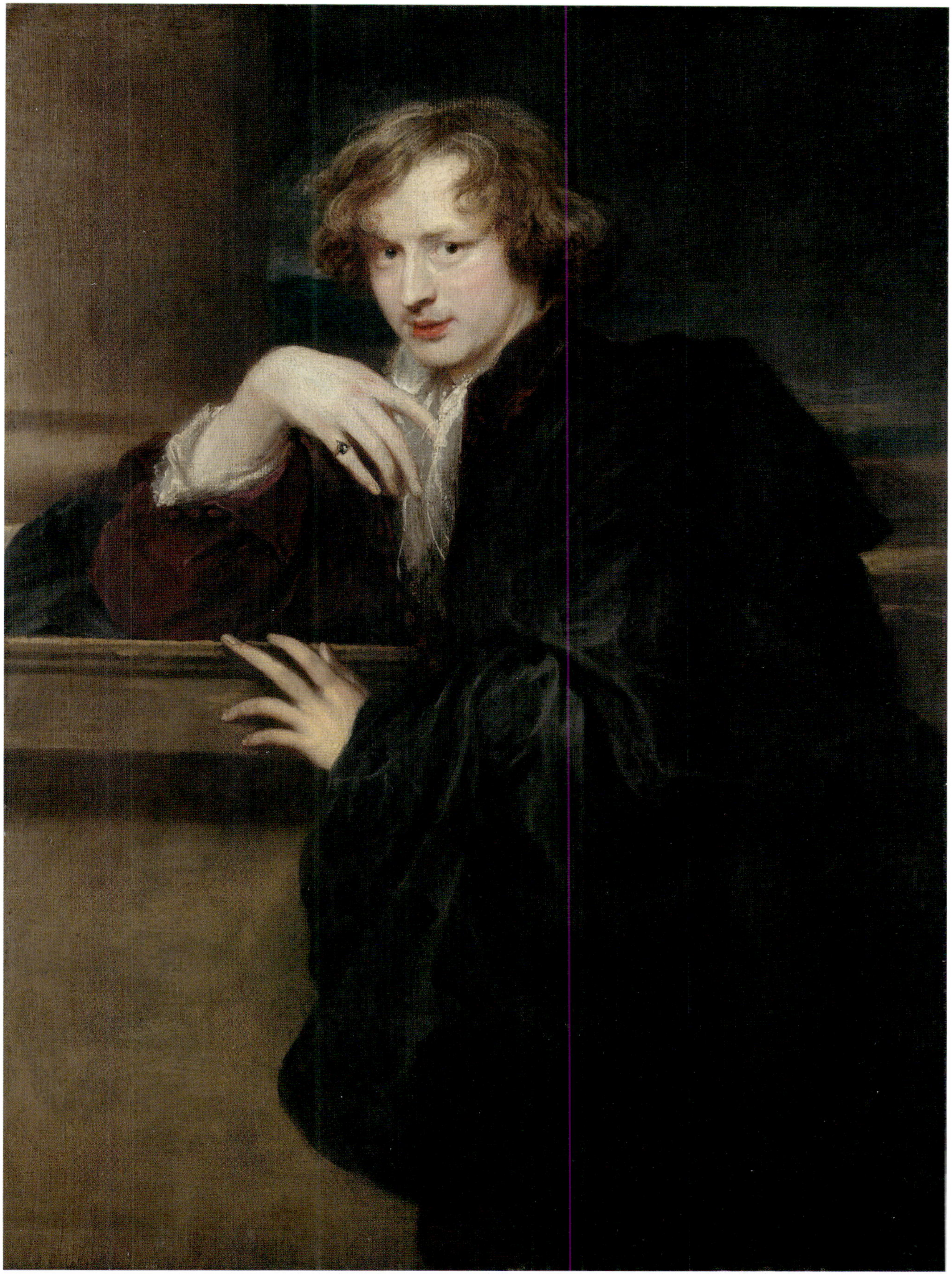

2 | Sir Anthony van Dyck
(1599–1641)

Emanuele Filiberto of Savoy

1624
Oil on canvas, 126 × 99.6 cm
Dulwich Picture Gallery, London
(DPG 173)

PROVENANCE

Emanuele Filiberto of Savoy, Prince of Oneglia and Viceroy of Sicily (1588–1624), Palermo; V. Donjeux; his sale, Paris, 29 April 1793 (lot 132), bought Desmarets; Noel Desenfans (1744–1807) and Sir Peter Francis Bourgeois (1753–1811), from at least 1795; bequeathed to Dulwich Picture Gallery, 1811.

According to Giovan Pietro Bellori's 1672 biography (2005, p. 217; 2009, p. 275), Van Dyck 'conceived a desire to move to Sicily where, as Prince Emanuele Filiberto of Savoy was viceroy at the time, he painted his portrait' ('venne desiderio ad Antonio di trasferirsi in Sicilia, dove trovandosi il principe Filiberto di Savoia allora viceré, fece il suo ritratto'). The anonymous French biographer recorded that 'Emanuele Filiberto of Savoy, viceroy of that island, and grand prior of Castille, called him to his court in 1624 and welcomed him with great honours. Van Dyck portrayed that prince and other patrons of that country' ('Emmanuel Philibert de Savoie, vice roi de cette île, et Grand-Prieur de Castille l'appela à sa cour en 1624 et lui fit un accueil très distingué. Vandyck peignit ce prince et quelques seigneurs de ce pays là,' Genoa 1997, p. 392). The commission of this portrait was the primary reason for Van Dyck's travel from Genoa to Palermo in the spring of 1624.

By 1795 the painting belonged to the art dealer and collector Noel Desenfans, who on 27 February of that year included the canvas in an auction sale of part of his collection in London, where it went unsold. In the auction catalogue the painting was described as 'the Portrait of General Schombergh'. It was subsequently recorded in the inventory of the collection of Desenfans's house, at 38–39 Charlotte Street, in the 'Upper Room, East Side of the Passage' as 'Port[rai]t Half length of the Duke D'Alva in armour' (Britton 1813). Gustav Friedrich Waagen and Anna Jameson identified the sitter as Archduke Albert, Governor of the Netherlands (Waagen 1838; Jameson 1842; Waagen 1854; Sparkes 1876; Richter and Sparkes 1880). Waagen even suggested the portrait may have been by Rubens rather than by Van Dyck. It was only in 1912 that Albert van de Put linked the painting with Bellori's account of Van Dyck's portrait of the viceroy. The identification was based on the discovery that the armour worn by the sitter was decorated with knots and crowns enclosing palm branches, both symbols usually associated with the Savoy family. Emanuele Filiberto is, in fact, wearing his magnificent Milanese armour, by the Maestro dal Castello, which survives in the Real Armería in Madrid (cat. 3).

The portrait was painted during the early summer of 1624, between Van Dyck's arrival in Palermo in the spring of that year and the viceroy's death on 3 August. The composition is based on the lost portrait of Emperor Charles V in armour by Titian, known through a copy painted by Rubens and an engraving by Lucas Vostermann. Van Dyck produced the perfect image of a seventeenth-century ruler, in which he combined martial prowess and foppish elegance. Emanuele Filiberto is portrayed wearing his armour for jousting on horseback, recognisable because of the lance rest on his breastplate. The armour is shown in its original colouring, with gilding and a blued background, which is almost entirely worn on the original.

It has been suggested that the portrait may have been connected to the negotiations of a marriage between Emanuele Filiberto and Maria Gonzaga, the daughter of Francesco IV and Margherita of Savoy (Baudi di Vesme 1885). She was the heir to the dukedom of Monferrato and the viceroy's father, Carlo Emanuele I, saw the wedding as a means to take over Gonzaga territories for the Savoy family. It is more likely, however, that rather than being a wedding portrait, the painting was commissioned simply as an official image of the viceroy. This was probably the picture that, according to Emanuele Filiberto's physician, Giovan Francesco Fiocchetto, was recorded in the Sala del Mosaico ('*cubiculo mosaico*' – fig. 14) of the Royal Palace in Palermo, and that, having fallen from the wall, was found on the floor of the room and interpreted by the viceroy as an ill omen, soon before his death from the plague.

There is no evidence as to where the portrait was between 1624 and 1793, when it appeared in an auction in Paris. Maria Beatrice Failla (2003, p. 69) suggested that the canvas may have passed to France via Piedmont. A portrait of Emanuele Filiberto is listed in Turin in the 1658 inventory of the collection of his brother, Tommaso di Carignano (Failla 2003, p. 69). This could be the same portrait 'of a man half length, in the taste of Van Dyck' ('d'un homme à demi corps dans le gout de Vandik') that appears in the *Catalogue des tableaux du cabinet de feu S.A.S. Monseigneur le prince de Carignan* in Paris in 1742. Another portrait of the viceroy arrived in Turin in 1736 from Genoa; Giovan Battista Cerruti was paid on 20 December of that year for having acquired a portrait of Emanuele Filiberto for the king, from a certain 'signor Garibaldi' ('A Gio. Batta. Cerruti in rimborso per aver pagato al sig. Garibaldi un quadro rappresentante l'effigie al naturale del fu serenissimo principe Filiberto di Savoia in suo vivente vice re di Sicilia acquistato da S.M. trasmesso a Torino, rec. 13 dicembre 1736, £ 200. 20 dicembre 1736', Archivio di Stato, Turin, Camerale Piemonte, art. 217, *Conti della tesoreria generale della Real Casa*, 1736, cap. 12, art. 74; Failla 2003, p. 86 n. 234).

A contemporary copy of the portrait was sold at auction at Christie's, London, 6 March 1936 (lot 151), and again at Christie's, London, 12 February 1954 (lot 50). According to Glück (1931) a small (63 × 52 cm) sketch of the head of the Dulwich portrait was in the Josephson collection in Stockholm, and he suggested that it could be an original sketch by Van Dyck; this is likely to be the same work that was previously in the Lamm collection in 1923 (Barnes 1986, p. 358, cat. C7). There are also references for a possible *modello* of the painting (104 × 74 cm – Barnes 1986, p. 359, cat. C8). As the whereabouts of both paintings are currently unknown, it is impossible to determine if these are by Van Dyck or, more likely, later copies.

SELECT BIBLIOGRAPHY

Britton 1813, p. 17; Waagen 1838, vol. 2, p. 380; Jameson 1842, pp. 478–79, cat. 218; Waagen 1854, vol. 2, p. 342; Sparkes 1876, p. 153, cat. 218; Richter and Sparkes 1880, pp. 53–54, cat. 218; Guiffrey 1882, p. 284, cat. 986; Baudi di Vesme 1885, pp. 25–26; Cust 1900, p. 243, cat. 115; Matranga 1908, p. 13; Schaeffer 1909, p. 436; Van De Put 1912; Van de Put 1914; Glück 1931, pp. 171, 538; Larsen 1980a, p. 117, cat. 438; Murray 1980, p. 55, cat. 173; Brown 1982, pp. 78,

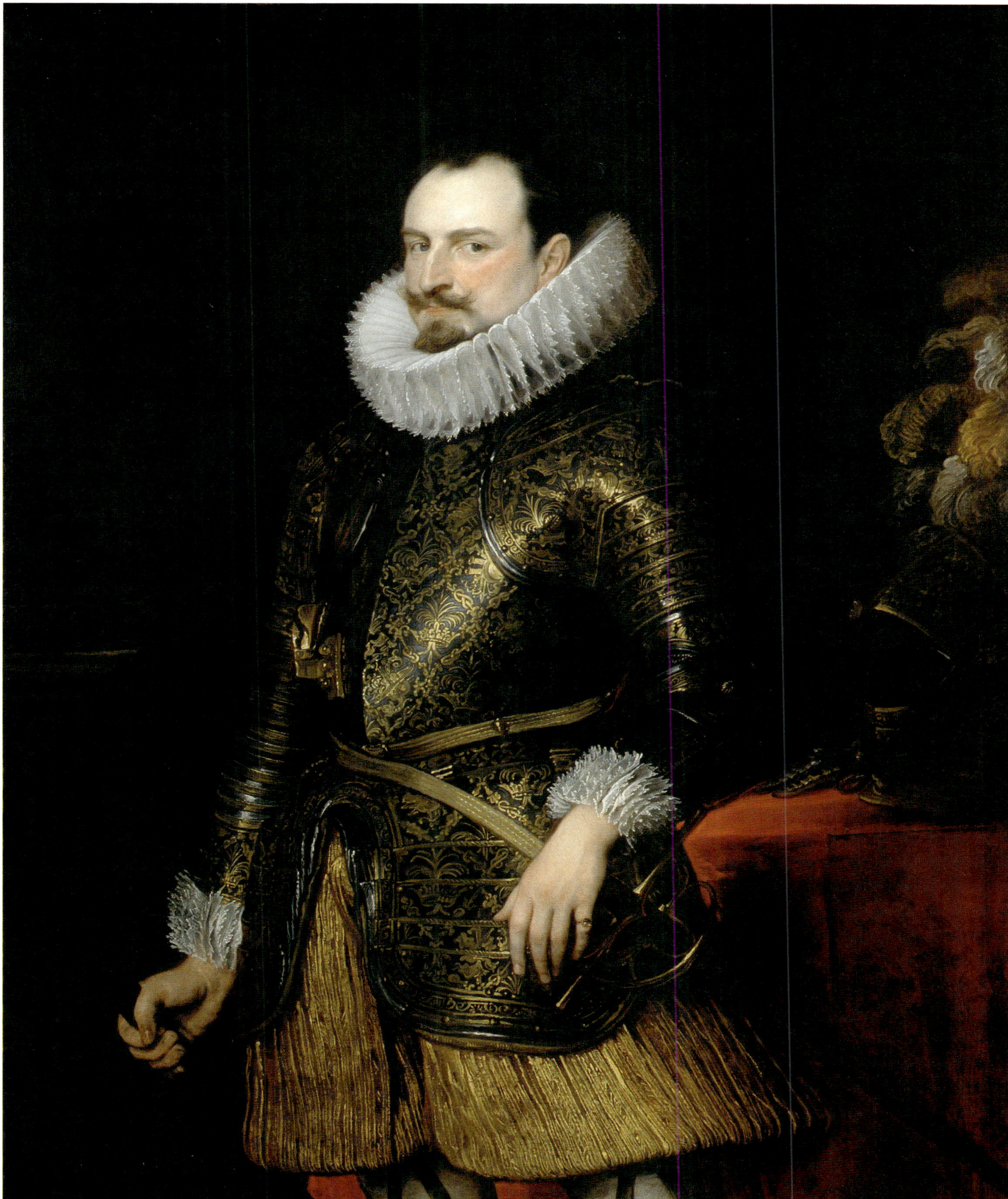

82–83; M. Ro-gers in Washington and Los Angeles 1985, pp. 52–53, cat. 6; Barnes 1986, pp. 14, 241–42, cat. 36; Boccia and Godoy 1987; Larsen 1988, p. 149, cat. 368; Abbate 1990, pp. 36–37; S.J. Barnes in Washington 1990, pp. 180–81, cat. 38; Beresford 1998, pp. 98–99, cat. 173; R. Oresko in Münster 1998, p. 39, cat. 37; I.A.C. Dejardin in Madrid and Bilbao 1999, pp. 112–13, cat. 23; C. Brown in London 1999a, pp. 172–73, cat. 35; Failla 2003, pp. 68–70; S.J. Barnes in Barnes, De Poorter, Millar, Vey 2004, pp. 200–03, cat. II.60; Abbate 2004, pp. 69–70; M.G. Bernardini in Milan 2004, pp. 124–25, 162, cat. 10; Bellori 2005, p. 217; M.B. Failla in Venaria Reale 2007, pp. 44–45, cat. 2.32; Bellori 2009, p. 275; X.F. Salomon in Washington 2009, p. 271, 273, cat. 67; Abbate 2011, pp. 85–86.

EXHIBITIONS

British Institution, London 1828, cat. 113; *Some Pictures from the Dulwich Gallery*, The National Gallery, London 1947, cat. 12; *Flemish Art, 1300–1700*, Royal Academy of Arts, London 1953–54, cat. 153; *Collection for a King: Old Master Paintings from the Dulwich Picture Gallery*, National Gallery of Art, Washington, and Los Angeles County Museum of Art, Los Angeles 1985–86, cat. 6; *Anthony van Dyck*, National Gallery of Art, Washington 1990–91, cat. 38; *1648. War and Peace in Europe*, Westfälisches Landesmuseum für Kunst und Kulturgeschichte, Münster 1998–99, cat. 37; *Obras Maestras de la Dulwich Picture Gallery*, Banco Bilbao Vizcaya, Madrid, and Museo de Bellas Artes, Bilbao 1999, cat. 23; *Van Dyck 1599–1641*, Koninklijk Museum voor Schone Kunsten, Antwerp, and Royal Academy of Arts, London 1999, cat. 35; *Anton van Dyck. Riflessi Italiani*, Palazzo Reale, Milan 2004, cat. 10; *La Reggia di Venaria e i Savoia. Arte, magnificenza e storia di una corte europea*, Reggia di Venaria Reale 2007, cat. 2.32; *The Art of Power. Royal Armor and Portraits from Imperial Spain*, National Gallery of Art, Washington 2009, cat. 67.

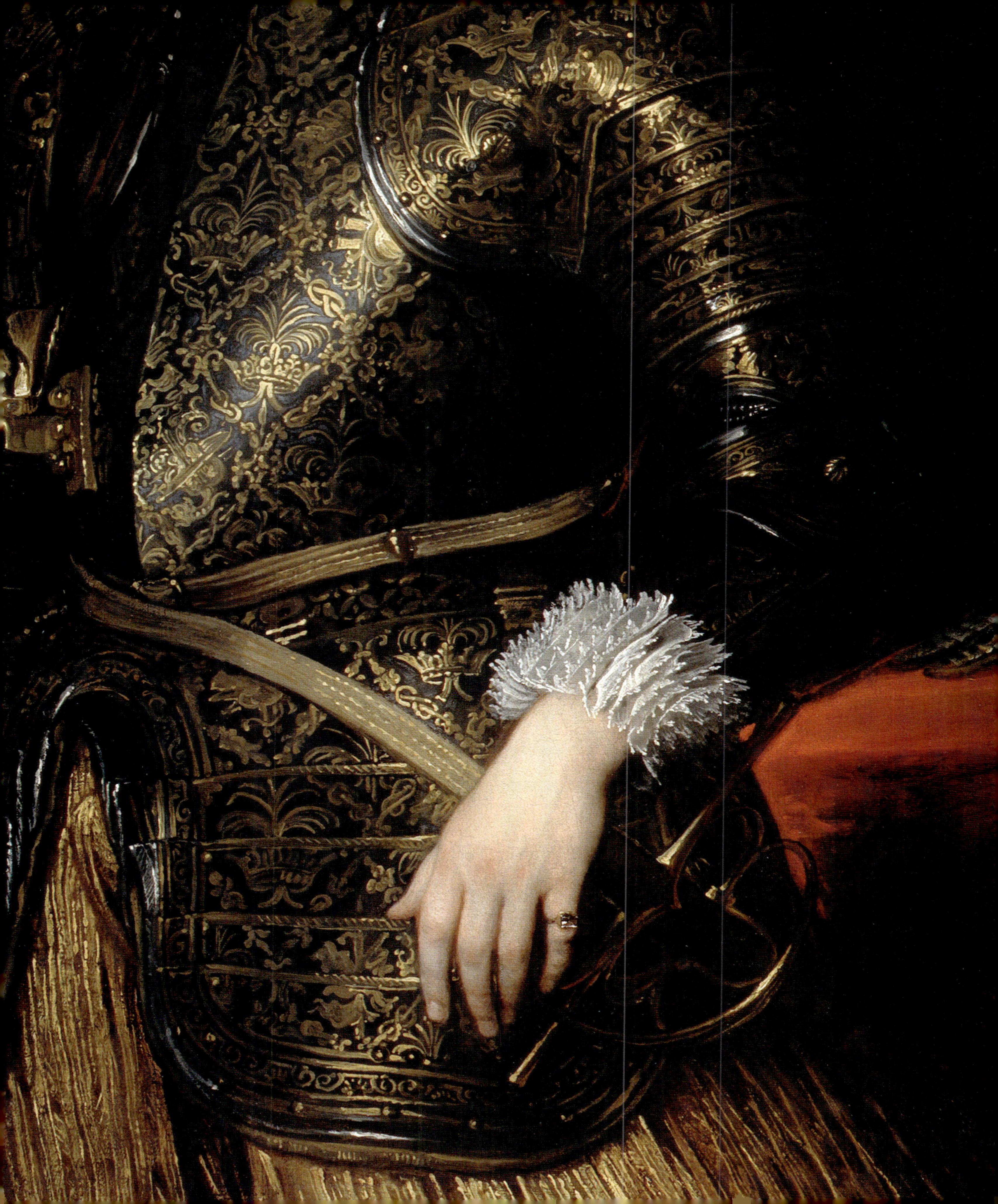

3 | Maestro dal Castello

(doc. 1590–1620)

Armour of Emanuele Filiberto of Savoy

c. 1606
Etched steel, partly gilt, height 180 cm
Patrimonio Nacional, Real Armería del Palacio Real de Madrid
(Inv. A. 360–368)

PROVENANCE

Emanuele Filiberto of Savoy (1588–1624); from 1625, Real Armería, Madrid.

The identity of the owner of this armour has been debated until the study of Lionello Boccia and José Godoy (1987). Achille Jubinal and Gaspard Sensi (1839) believed it belonged to Saint Ignatius of Loyola, Antonio Martínez del Romero (1849) gave it to Duke Emanuele Filiberto of Savoy (1528–80), while Juan Bautista de Valencia de Don Juan (1898) identified it with the armour of Filippo Emanuele of Savoy (1586–1605). The connection to Filippo Emanuele has proved particularly popular until recent times (Cervini 2007). Boccia and Godoy, however, have established without any doubt that this garniture was designed for Emanuele Filiberto of Savoy, Viceroy of Sicily, and it is the one depicted by Van Dyck in his portrait of the viceroy, now at Dulwich Picture Gallery (cat. 2). The armour is described in the 1624 inventory of Emanuele Filiberto's collection ('de campo abierto de a cavallo doradas con la granadura de palmas y coronas y tiene una celada y peto y un bra[z]cal y una manopla de respeto y sirven de tornear a piè', Failla 2003, pp. 51, 77 n. 105) and in later inventories of the Real Armería in Madrid.

The armour is actually a garniture, composed of elements for different types of the tournament, jousting on horseback ('*di rincontro*') and foot combat ('*campo aperto*'). It has, therefore, two breastplates and two helmets, one for each type of tournament (in the Van Dyck portrait, Emanuele Filiberto is shown wearing the horseback one). The elements were originally gilt on a blued background, now mostly worn, but the original, splendid, effect can be seen in the Van Dyck painting. The Savoia emblems of the knots ('*nodo Savoia*') and palms and crowns are visible throughout the garniture, on the two armours, and also on the two hand defences for lances (vamplates) and the horse's head defence (shaffron).

Three of the children of Duke Carlo Emanuele I – Filippo Emanuele, Vittorio Amedeo and Emanuele Filiberto – were at the Spanish court between June 1603 and August 1606. Filippo Emanuele, often mistakenly identified as the owner of the armour, died of smallpox in Valladolid on 9 February 1605. It is likely that this garniture was made for Emanuele Filiberto upon his return to Turin in 1606, possibly even as a gift from his uncle, King Philip III of Spain. After Emanuele Filiberto's death, his body was returned to Spain, on a ship that sailed from Palermo on 2 September 1625; the armour was among the viceroy's personal effects that were sent to Spain on the same ship. As illustrated in Van Dyck's portrait, the armour was originally worn with a sword, now lost. The Armería inventories, however, also register two guns that belonged to Emanuele Filiberto, one of which – a triple-barrel gun – still survives (fig. 37 – also described in the 1624 inventory of the viceroy's possessions, see Failla 2003, pp. 52, 78 n. 113).

The author of Emanuele Filiberto's particularly rich and highly decorated garniture is the still anonymous Maestro dal Castello, whose name derives from signing his armours with a small castle with three towers, usually on the neck of the breastplate. He is documented as working in Milan from around 1590 to 1620, and his work survives in the Armeria Reale in Turin, the Castello Sforzesco and Museo Poldi Pezzoli in Milan, and the Metropolitan Museum of Art in New York. Most of the maestro's armours were decorated with Savoia emblems, suggesting a strong relationship with this specific dynasty. Stylistically, the Maestro dal Castello is particularly close to the '*armaiolo regio*' Pompeo della Cesa, and it has even been suggested that he may be identified with his son Guidalberto, or Vitalberto.

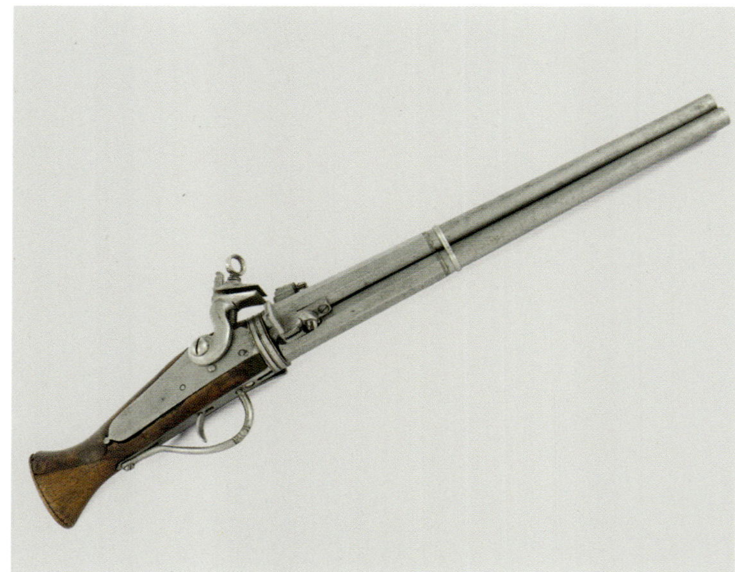

37 | Gun of Emanuele Filiberto of Savoy. Patrimonio Nacional, Real Armería, Madrid

SELECT BIBLIOGRAPHY

Jubinal and Sensi 1839, vol. 2, plate XIX, fig. 1, plate XX bis, figs. 6–7; Martínez del Romero 1849, pp. 13–14, 47, 73, 184–85, cat. 2469; Valencia de Don Juan 1898, pp. 107–08, cat. A. 360–68; Boccia and Coelho 1967, pp. 473–74; Boccia and Godoy 1987; Godoy 1987, pp. 16–20; Failla 2003, pp. 51–52, 77–78; F. Cervini in Venaria Reale 2007, p. 43, cat. 2.30; A. Soler del Campo in Washington 2009, pp. 191, 270, cat. 66; A. Soler del Campo in Madrid 2010, pp. 75, 79.

EXHIBITIONS

La Reggia di Venaria e i Savoia. Arte, magnificenza e storia di una corte europea, Reggia di Venaria Reale 2007, cat. 2.30; *The Art of Power. Royal Armor and Portraits from Imperial Spain*, National Gallery of Art, Washington 2009, cat. 66.

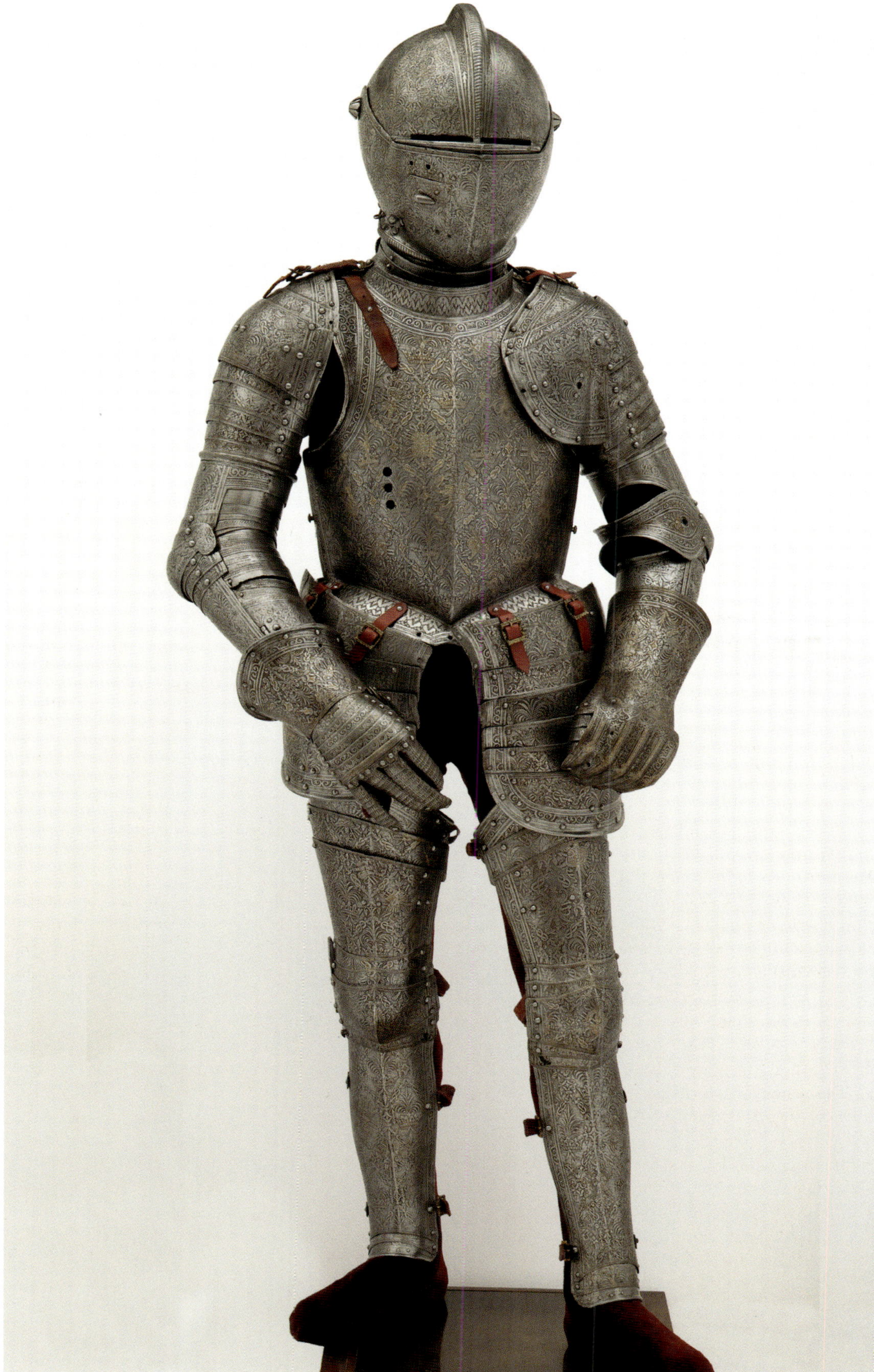

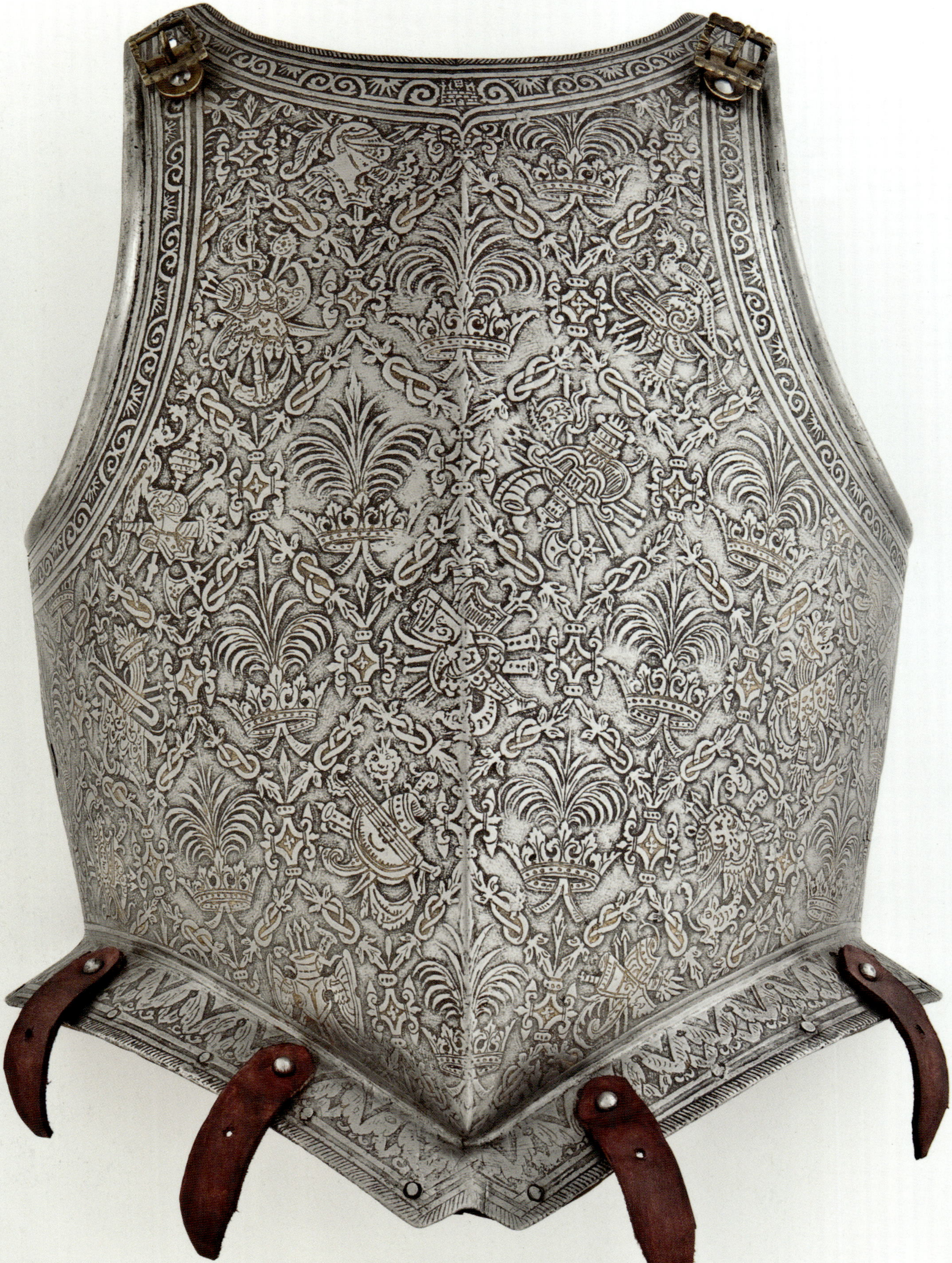

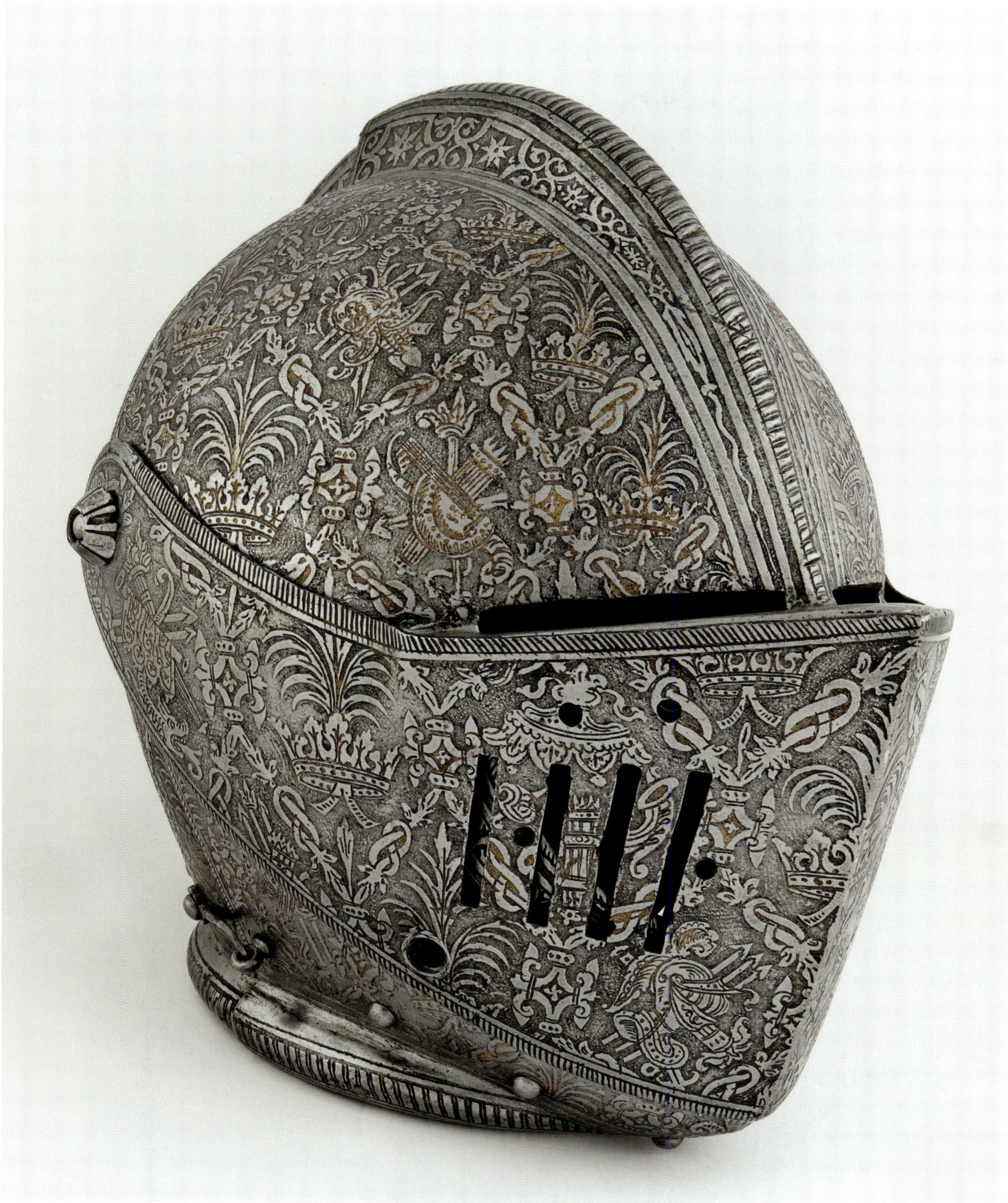

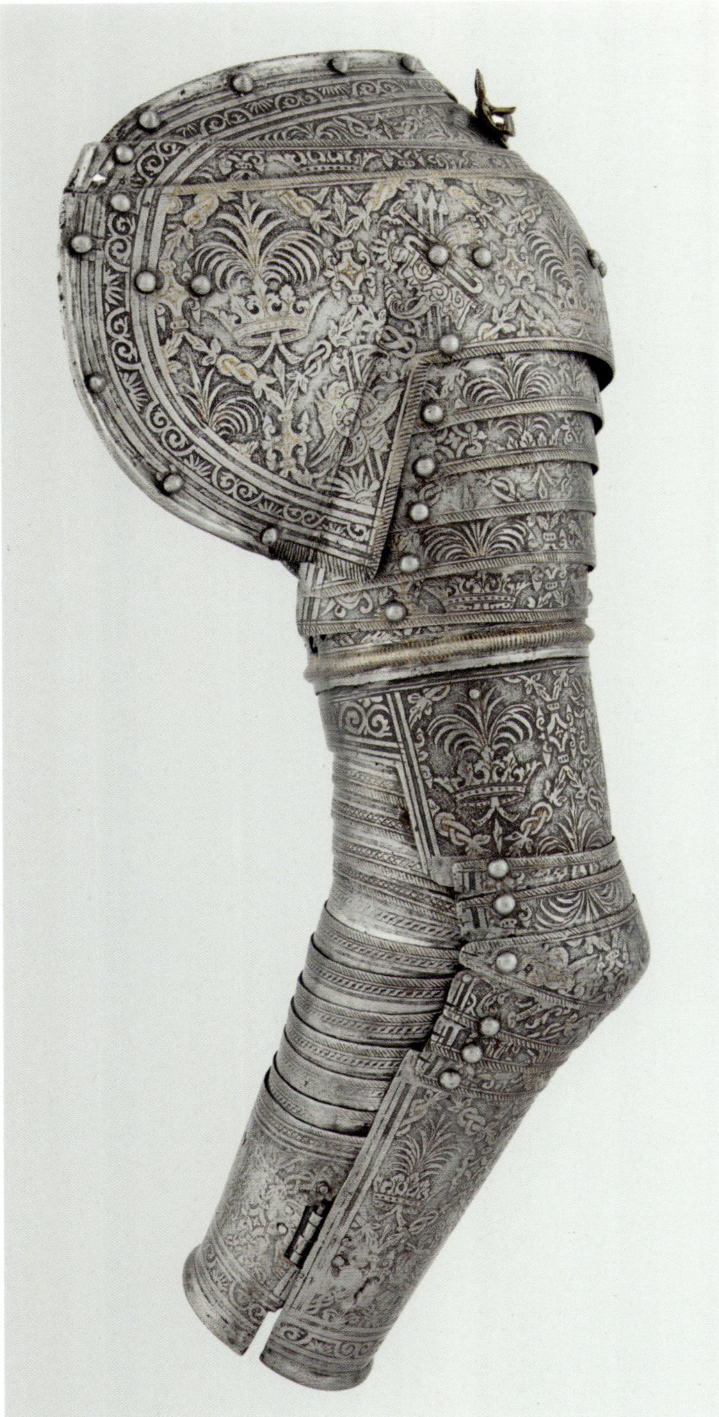

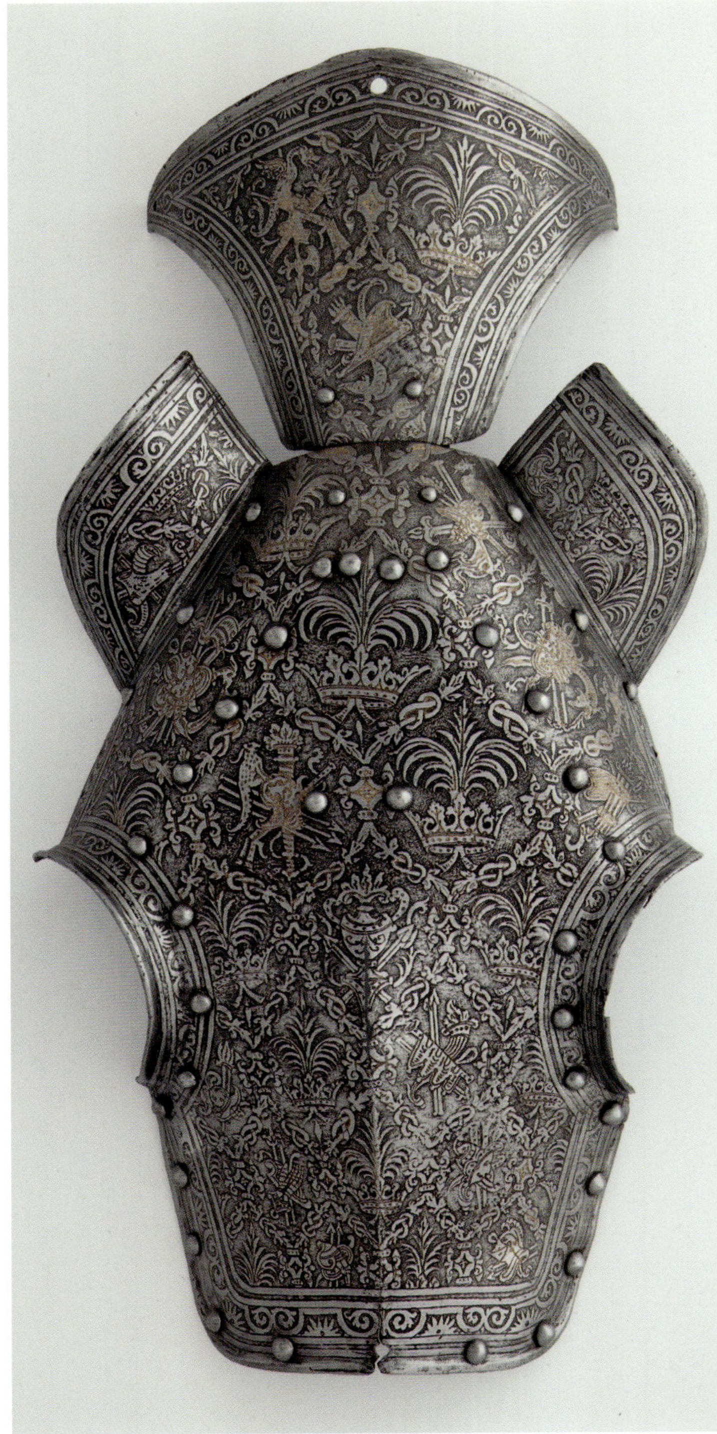

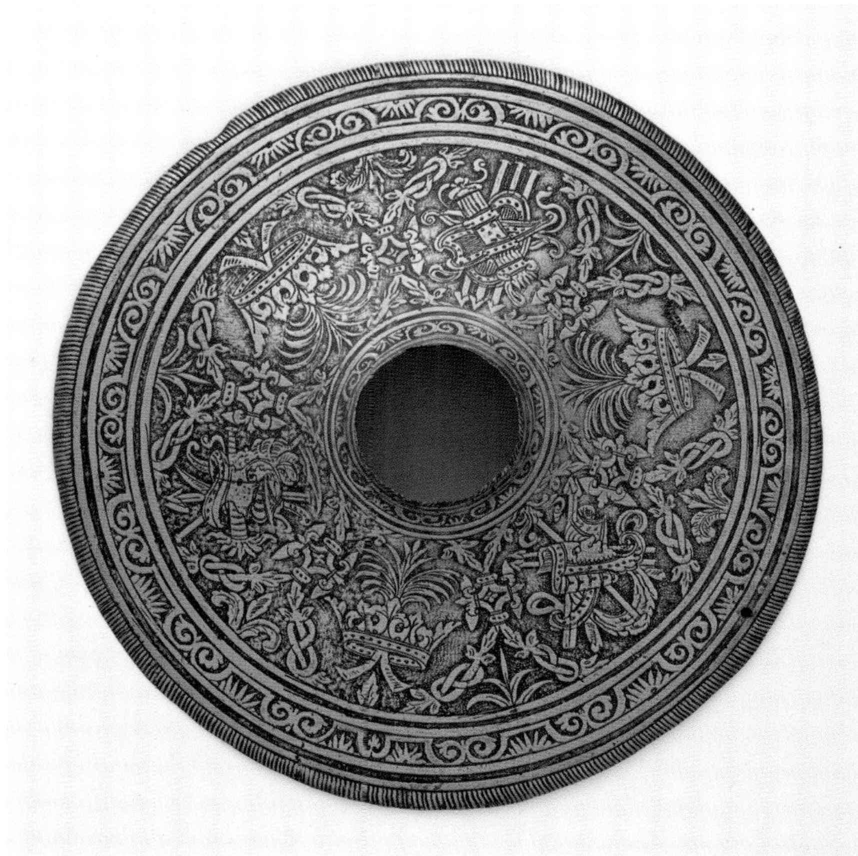

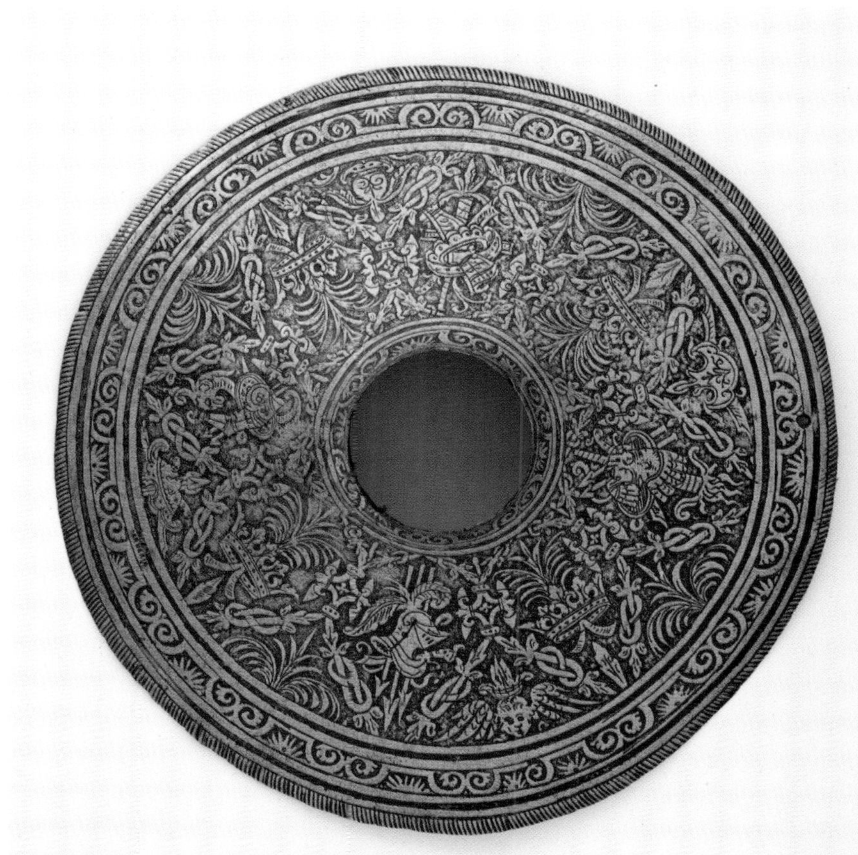

4 | Attributed to Tommaso Carlone
(d. 1667)

Emanuele Filiberto of Savoy

c. 1635
Marble, 96 × 66.5 × 37.5 cm
Galleria Sabauda, Turin
(Inv. 20/720)

PROVENANCE
Collection of Savoy family; Galleria Sabauda, Turin, since at least 1865.

The marble bust is identified as a portrait of Duke Emanuele Filiberto of Savoy 'il Muto' (1628–1709) in the 1865 manuscript inventory of the Galleria Sabauda in Turin (Gabrielli 1971). The armour worn by the sitter in the bust is clearly earlier than the mid- to late seventeenth century, and Pompeo Litta (1872) rightly recognised the man portrayed as Emanuele Filiberto, Viceroy of Sicily. Until recently there has been some confusion on the identity of the sitter, and Gabrielli (1971) described him as Duke Vittorio Amedeo I. It is clear, however, by comparing the Van Dyck portrait of Emanuele Filiberto (cat. 2) with the bust, and by recognising the cross of Malta on the breastplate of the armour, that this is a portrait of the Viceroy of Sicily. The bust is accompanied by two others of his brothers, Duke Vittorio Amedeo I (wrongly identified by Gabrielli 1971 as another brother, Tommaso di Carignano), and Cardinal Maurizio.

The authorship of the bust has been little studied. Generally it has been catalogued as anonymous (Litta 1872; Gabrielli 1971), or as the work of an unknown sculptor of the Luganese school (Pinto and Di Macco 1991; Spantigati 2000). Failla (2003) attributed the bust to Tommaso Carlone (for whom, see Tamburini 1977). Carlone was born in Rovio, near Lugano, and came from a family of sculptors. He travelled and worked around Italy in the first half of the seventeenth century. He is documented in Genoa around 1600, in Rome in 1606 and in Milan in 1632. He was in Turin, working for the Savoy family around 1633–35 and again between 1653 and his death in 1667. In Turin Carlone restored ancient sculptures, and produced works for palaces and churches. He decorated the chapel of the Madonna del Buon Soccorso and the high altar of San Francesco di Paola for Cardinal Maurizio of Savoy, Emanuele Filiberto's brother. It is likely that this is a posthumous bust, made after Emanuele Filiberto's death in 1624, and during Carlone's first Torinese sojourn. Carlone is known to have carved another image of the viceroy; the 1645 inventory of Giacomo Francesco Arpino (1608–84), personal doctor to Cardinal Maurizio of Savoy, lists 'a portrait of the Most Serene Prince Emanuele Filiberto of Savoy also in an oval in plaster in low relief, and by the hand of the above said Carlone, 2 *piedi* high' ('un ritratto del Serenissimo Prencipe Emanuel Filiberto di Savoia anche in un'ovato di gezzo a basso rilievo, e di mano del sudetto Carlone d'altezza piedi 2'), which served as a pendant to another oval low-relief with the portrait of Cardinal Maurizio (Cifani and Monetti 1990, p. 68).

SELECT BIBLIOGRAPHY
Litta 1872, plate XXXVIII; Gabrielli 1971, pp. 266–67, cat. 20; Pinto and Di Macco 1991, p. 34, cat. 20; C.E. Spantigati in Astrua and Spantigati 2000, p. 67; Failla 2003, pp. 70, 87 n. 247.

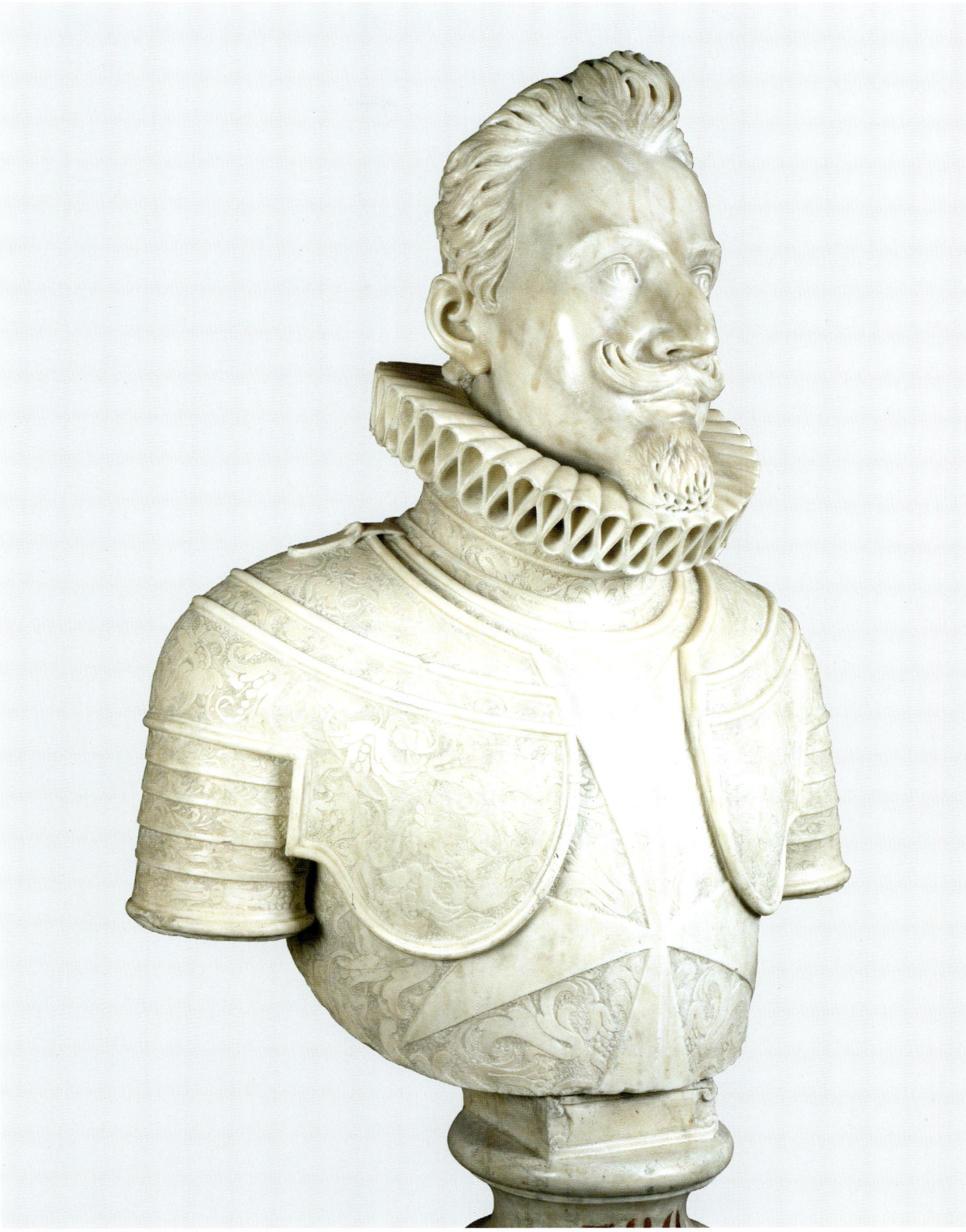

8

Ritratto della Sig.ra Sofonisma pittricia fatto dal vivo in

l'anno 1624 li 12 di Julio. l'età di essa 96 havendo ancora

et il cervello prontissimo, cortesissima. Et sebene per la ve

mancava la vesta. hebbe con tutto ciò gusto di mettere gli qua

d'essa et con gran stenta mettendo il naso sopra il

discernere qualche poco et ~~piglio~~ piglio gran

quel modo, facendo il retratto de es

diversi advertimenti non dovendo

troppo alto, acciò che le om

e della vecchiaia non diven

ando, et molti altri buo

ne ancora con to parte della

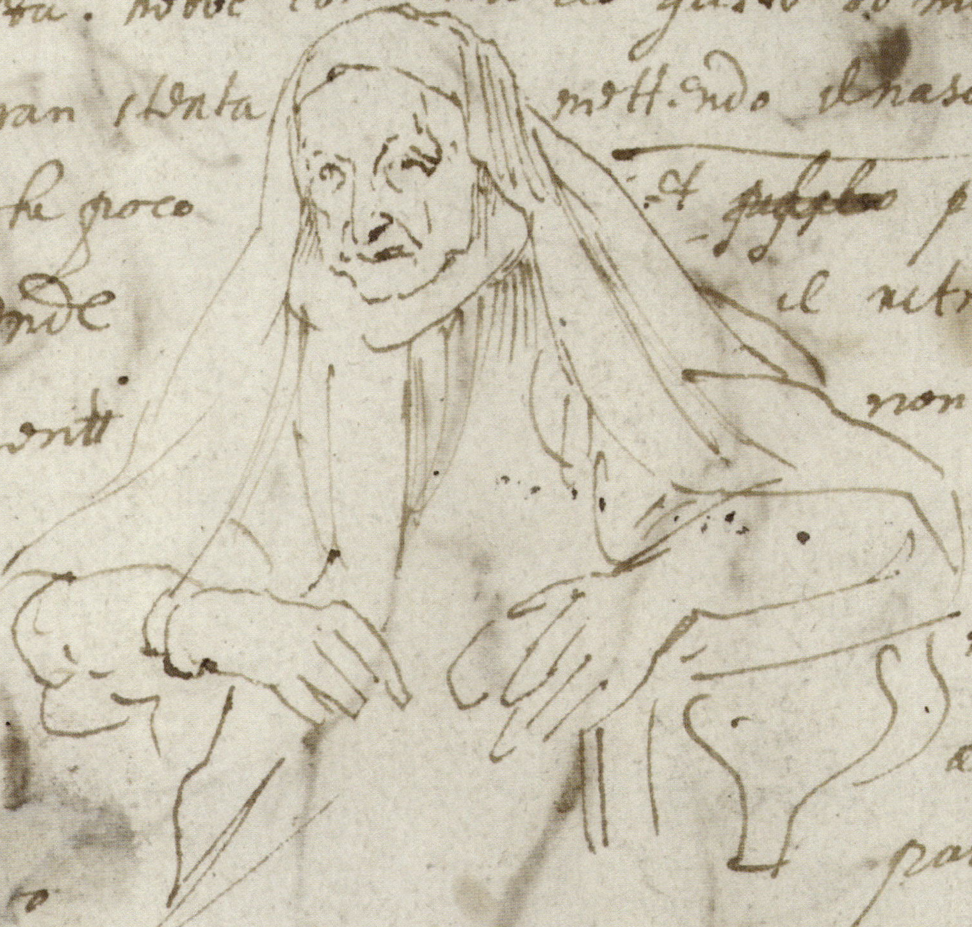

er la quale si conobbe ch'era pittora di natura mi

t. la pena maggiore che hebbe era per mancamento

~~[illegible]~~ non poter più dipingere. la mano era ancora fer

rdinbula nessuna.

Portraiture: Sofonisba Anguissola and Desiderio Segno

5 | Sir Anthony van Dyck
(1599–1641)

Italian Sketchbook – Sofonisba Anguissola

1624
Pen and ink on paper, 235 × 180 mm
The British Museum, London
(BM 1957.1214.207)

Inscribed: '*Ritratto della Sig[no]ra Sofonisma pittricia fatto dal viva in Pal[erm]o l'anno 1624 li 12 di Julio, l'età di essa 96 havendo ancora la memoria et il serverllo prontissimo, cortesissima, et sebene perla vecciaia la mancava la vista, hebbe con tutto cio gusto de mettere gli quadri avanti ad essa et con gran stenta mettendo il naso sopra il quadro, venne a discernere qualche poco et piglio gran piacere ancora in quel modo, facende il ritratto de essa, mi diede diversi advertimenti non devendo pigliar il lume troppo alto, accio che le ombre nelle ruge della vecciaia non diventassero troppo grande, et molti altri buoni discorsi come ancora conto parte della vita di essa per la quale se conobbe che era pittora de natura et miraculosa et la pena magiore che hebbe era per mancamento di vista non poter più dipingere, la mano era ancora ferma senza tremula nessuna*'

PROVENANCE

Sir Anthony van Dyck (1599–1641); Sir Peter Lely (1618–80); Prosper Henricus Lankrink (1628–92); Hugh Howard; his brother the Bishop of Elphin; in family of Earls of Wicklow by descent; Dukes of Devonshire, by 1735 (disappeared from collection at an unknown date in the eighteenth century); Samuel William Reynolds (1773–1835); sold to George James Welbore Agar-Ellis, 1st Baron Dover (1797–1833), 1830; his son Henry Agar-Ellis, 3rd Viscount Clifden (1825–66); his son Henry George Agar-Ellis, 4th Viscount Clifden (1863–95); Christie's, London, 6 May 1893 (lot 36); bought Deprez; Charles Fairfax Murray (1849–1919); Herbert F. Cook (1868–1939); returned to Duke of Devonshire; accepted *in lieu* of inheritance tax and allocated by H.M. Treasury to the British Museum, 1957.

While travelling around Italy, between 1621 and 1627, Van Dyck carried with him a small quarto volume in which he drew about two hundred images as a visual diary. The *Italian Sketchbook* contains mostly representations of works of art that Van Dyck saw and recorded in Italy, and a few depictions of people taken from life; on one occasion, he drew sitters for portraits he was painting, Sir Robert and Lady Shirley in Rome in 1622. The painter was particularly interested in the composition of the works he recorded, but he also annotated them with comments on colours and on the quality of the objects. He recorded the way in which light was depicted and documented costumes with special attention. Most of the artworks drawn by Van Dyck were Old Master paintings, by artists such as Leonardo da Vinci, Giorgione, Sebastiano del Piombo, Raphael, Paolo Veronese, Parmigianino, Marcantonio Raimondi, Albrecht Dürer and Giovan Battista Moroni, but he was also interested in works by contemporary painters like Annibale Carracci, Guercino and Orazio Gentileschi. The artist that was single-handedly most often copied by Van Dyck was Titian, and in the *Sketchbook* he recorded many of his most celebrated paintings, including the *Pala Pesaro* (Santa Maria Gloriosa dei Frari, Venice), *Sacred and Profane Love* (Galleria Borghese, Rome), the *Venus of Urbino* (Galleria degli Uffizi, Florence), the *Portrait of Pope Paul III and his Family* (Museo di Capodimonte, Naples), and numerous other portraits. Copies were also made after drawings, prints and sculptures. In general antiquity does not seem to have interested Van Dyck particularly and there are few drawings of ancient sculptures, and one very careful study of the so-called *Nozze Aldobrandini* (Musei Vaticani, Rome), an ancient fresco.

The *Sketchbook* was preserved in Van Dyck's workshop and he presumably used it as a source of inspiration and as a pattern book throughout his career. It was with the painter when he died in London in 1641, and it then passed on to another artist, Sir Peter Lely, and to his assistant, Prosper Henricus Lankrink. The *Sketchbook* was then acquired by Hugh Howard, who is believed to have strengthened many of the chalk drawings by Van Dyck in the book with ink. By the late 18th century the *Italian Sketchbook* was in the collection of the Dukes of Devonshire, from where it went missing. It reappeared in 1830 when the engraver Samuel William Reynolds sold it to Baron Dover, who had the volume bound in its present red plush cover. By the time the *Sketchbook* reached Herbert Cook, through Charles Fairfax Murray, it was discovered that this was the volume that had gone missing from the Devonshire collection and it was promptly returned to Chatsworth. It was acquired by the British Museum in 1957.

Few of the pages in the *Sketchbook* relate to Van Dyck's stay in Palermo in 1624–25. There are drawings of a witch (fig. 8) and of actors and acrobats (figs. 6–7) in the streets of the city. In one of the first pages, he jotted down the name of Fabrizio Valguarnera 'Dottore in Palermo' (fig. 21). The most significant sketch from the Sicilian period is the portrait of the aged painter Sofonisba Anguissola. Van Dyck represented her in the middle of the sheet, sitting on a large armchair, her arms resting on it, and posing for the young Flemish painter who was drawing her. The sketch was probably made from life, while Van Dyck was conversing with Sofonisba. He subsequently added, in his own hand and in Italian, a detailed account of the visit: 'portrait of the painter Signora Sofonisba, done from life in Palermo in the year 1624, on 12 July: her age being 96 years, still with her memory and brain most quick, and most kind, and although she has lost her sight because of her old age, she enjoyed to have paintings put in front of her, and with great effort by placing her nose close to the picture, she could make out a little of it, and she took great pleasure in that. As I was doing her portrait, she gave me various recommendations, of not to take the light too high, so that the shadows in the wrinkles of old age should not be too strong, and many other good suggestions. And she also told me part of the story of her life, from which I learnt that she was a painter from nature and a miraculous one, and her greatest misfortune was that she could not paint any longer because of her lack of eyesight: even though her hand was still firm and with no tremor whatsoever.' This is a unique instance in the entire *Sketchbook* where Van Dyck recorded an autobiographical event. It is a vivid account of the encounter between two celebrated portrait painters from different eras, but also the poignant description of an older artist passing her knowledge and instructions on to a younger man. Van Dyck's reverence towards Sofonisba is evident in the fact itself that he recorded their conversation in such detail, but the text also gives us a glimpse of Anguissola's own interest and desire to share her experience with the promising young foreign painter.

SELECT BIBLIOGRAPHY

Antwerp 1899, p. 65, cat. 115; Cust 1902; Adriani 1940; Egger 1942; Tietze-Conrat 1950; Brown 1982, pp. 64–73, 82–84; C. Brown in New York and Fort Worth 1991, pp. 30–33; M. Gregori in Cremona, Vienna and Washington 1994, pp. 32, 42; Sacchi 1994, pp. 166, 169; S. Ferino-Pagden in Washington 1995, p. 97; C. Brown in London 1999a, pp. 22–25; Ekserdjian 2000; Jaffé 2001; McGrath 2001; Jaffé 2002, vol. 1, pp. 70–127; V. Abbate in Milan 2004, p. 71.

EXHIBITIONS

Van Dijk Tentoonstelling, Koninklijk Museum voor Schone Kunsten, Antwerp 1899, cat. 115; *Shah 'Abbas. The Remaking of Iran*, The British Museum, London 2009, cat. 18.

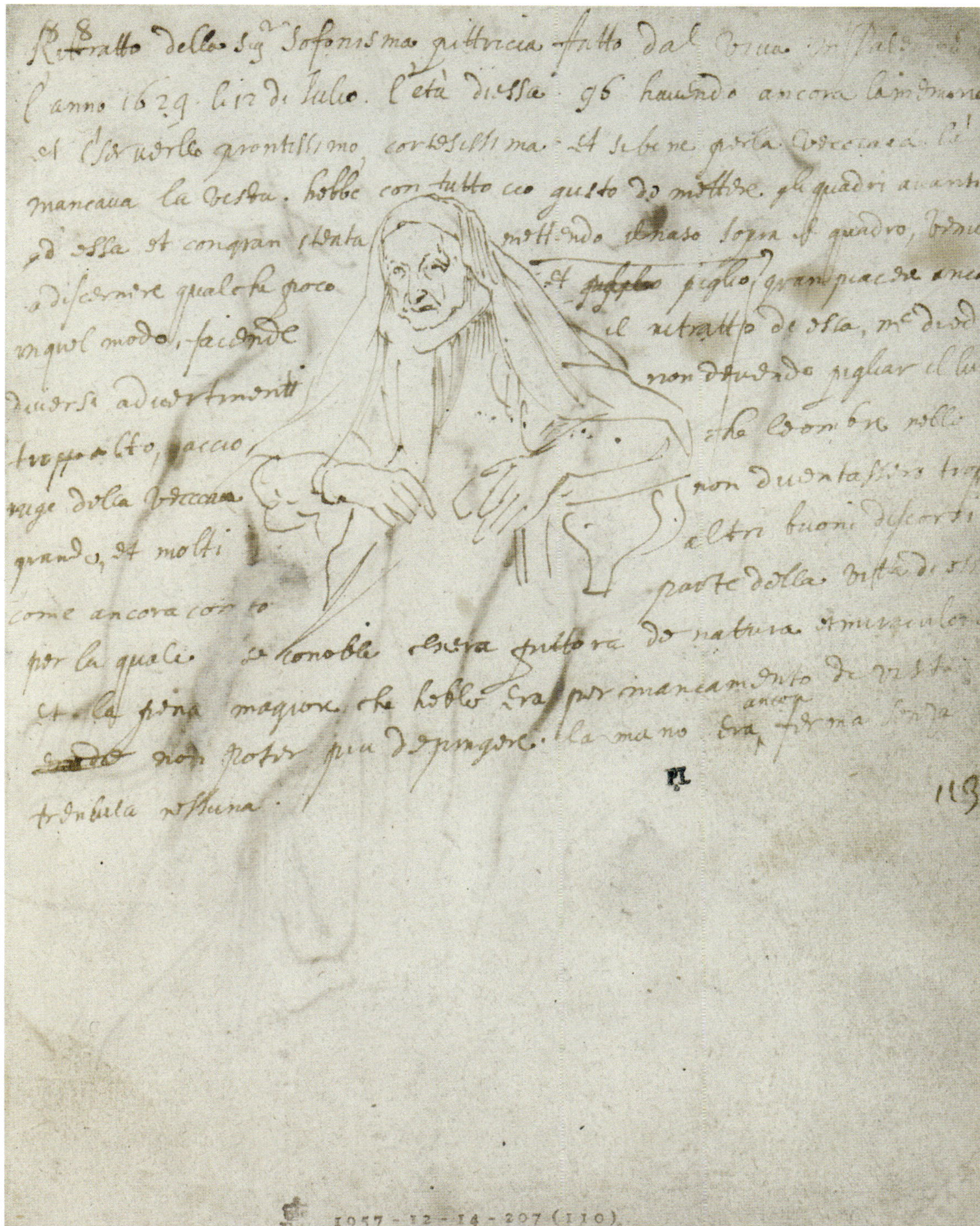
BM
1957-12-14-207 (110)

6 | Sir Anthony van Dyck
(1599–1641)

Sofonisba Anguissola

1624
Oil on canvas, 42 × 33.5 cm
Sackville Collection, Knole
(Inv. S.KNO.P.192)

PROVENANCE

Possibly brought by Arabella Diana, 3rd Duchess of Dorset (d. 1825), daughter and co-heiress of Sir Charles Cope, to Knole, Sevenoaks, Kent; thence by descent to Lord Sackville at Knole.

The small canvas probably entered the collection at Knole, through the 3rd Duchess of Dorset, before her death in 1825. It was described as a portrait of Catherine Fitzgerald, Countess of Desmond, who died in 1636 (Bridgman 1817; Brady 1839). Oliver Millar in 1969 connected for the first time the painting with Van Dyck's drawing of Sofonisba Anguissola, made on 12 July 1624 in his *Italian Sketchbook* (cat. 5). The features of the sitter in the Sackville portrait are the same as those of Sofonisba in the British Museum sketch; she wears the same outfit, the black dress, with white collar and veil. The painting clearly derives from the drawing in the *Sketchbook*.

Millar's attribution of the Knole portrait to Van Dyck has been rejected (Larsen 1980a did not include it in his catalogue of Van Dyck's paintings) and questioned, suggesting that it may be a copy after a lost original (Abbate 2004 and 2011). Because of the canvas's poor condition it is difficult to attribute conclusively the portrait to the artist, but Miller's proposal is in general convincing. It is likely that Van Dyck painted this canvas immediately after meeting Sofonisba in July 1624, basing the composition on the drawing he sketched of her from life. In the *Sketchbook* Van Dyck wrote about 'paintings put in front of her [Sofonisba]' ('mettere gli quadri avanti ad essa') and about 'doing her portrait' ('facende il ritratto de essa'). There is no evidence as to what paintings Van Dyck showed the aged painter in July 1624; it is also unclear what 'portrait' he made of her from life. Most likely, this was the drawing in the *Italian Sketchbook*, and it seems reasonable that the Knole portrait was based on the sketch and painted in Van Dyck's studio subsequently.

The surface of the painting is abraded, leaving only a faint impression of how powerful the painting must have originally been. The lack of cusping on all four sides of the canvas demonstrates that it was cut down, and that this is a fragment of a larger portrait. Possibly the painting was originally a half-length following exactly the composition of the *Sketchbook* drawing, with Sofonisba sitting in a chair. X-ray analysis has revealed important changes in the shape and size of the sitter's white collar.

SELECT BIBLIOGRAPHY

Bridgman 1817, pp. 33–34; Brady 1839, pp. 15–16; Millar 1969, p. 417; Jaffé 2002, p. 119; Abbate 2004, p. 71; S.J. Barnes in Barnes, De Poorter, Millar, Vey 2004, p. 171, cat. II.27; Abbate 2011, pp. 87–88.

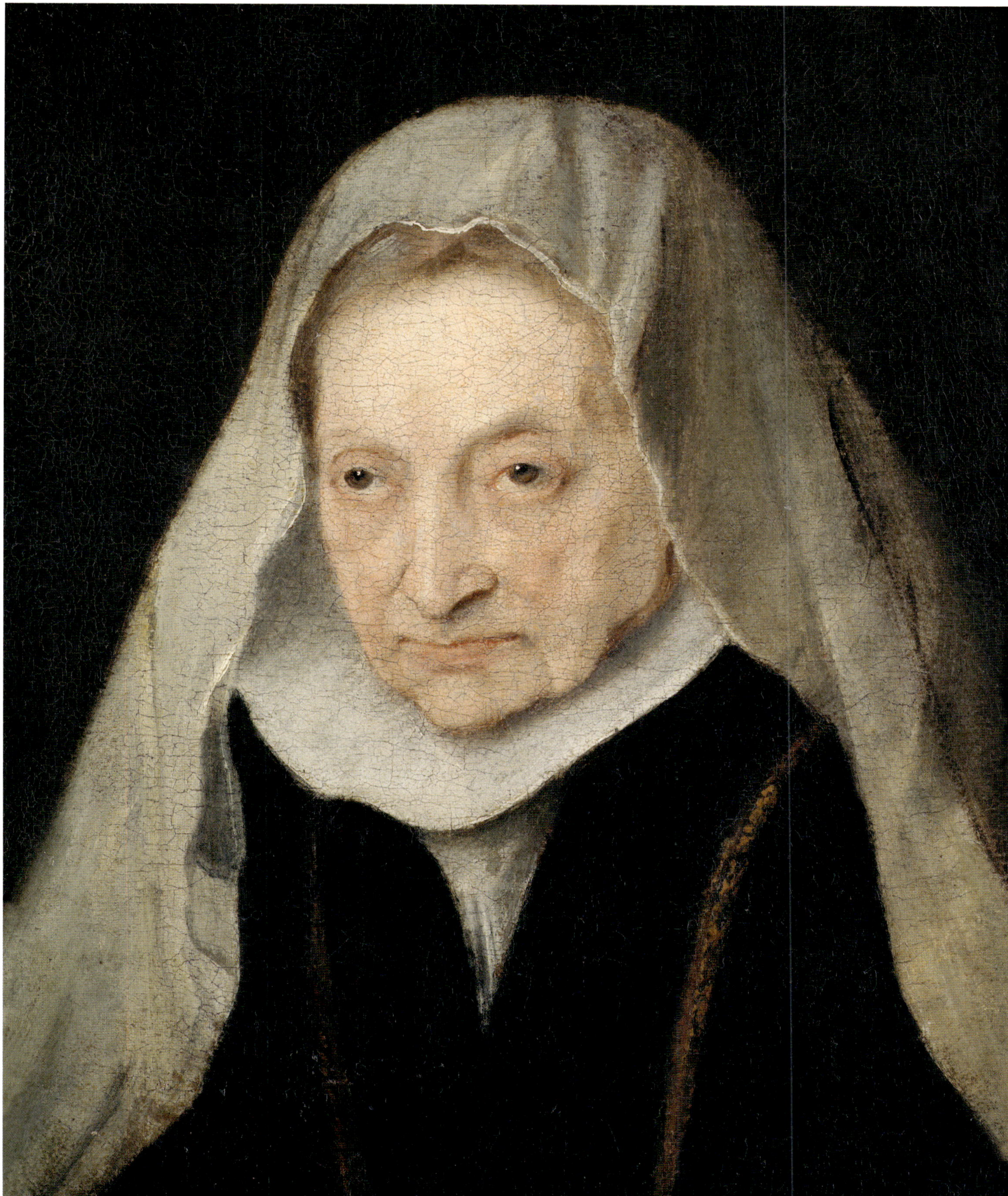

7 | Style of Sir Anthony van Dyck
(1599–1641)

Sofonisba Anguissola (?) on her Deathbed

After 1625
Oil on canvas, 52 × 72 cm
Galleria Sabauda, Turin
(Inv. 304)

PROVENANCE
Private collection, Palermo, by 1902; Simonetti collection, Rome; Riccardo Gualino (1879–1964), Turin, by 1926; Gualino gift to Galleria Sabauda, 1930.

Lionel Cust, in 1902, writing about the drawing of Sofonisba Anguissola in Van Dyck's *Italian Sketchbook* (cat. 5), noticed that 'a painting somewhat resembling this drawing by Van Dyck has lately been discovered at Palermo, and attributed to Van Dyck'. According to Lionello Venturi (1926) this was the same painting that had passed through the Simonetti collection in Rome and was by that date in the collection of Riccardo Gualino in Turin.

The picture portrays an aged woman on her deathbed, holding a rosary in her hands. Venturi described the 'calm penumbra, the slow and by now timid pulse of life' ('questa penombra calma, in questo pulsare lento e ormai timido di vita'). She has traditionally been identified as Sofonisba Anguissola. The physical similarity between the woman and Van Dyck's portraits of Sofonisba in the *Italian Sketchbook* and in the Knole portrait (cat. 6) is generic. Sofonisba Anguissola died on 16 November 1625 in Palermo, and as Van Dyck is last documented in Sicily in September of that year, it is unlikely that he was in the city when Sofonisba died. Stylistically the Turin canvas seems to be far from Van Dyck's manner of painting. In composition the painting is not dissimilar from Van Dyck's portrait of Venetia Stanley, Lady Digby, on her deathbed, painted in 1633 (Dulwich Picture Gallery, London, see London 1995a and O. Millar in Barnes, De Poorter, Millar, Vey 2004, pp. 506–07, cat. IV.97 – fig. 38). In both pictures a woman is shown half-length in a bed, diagonally placed across the picture plane, with her head resting on a large pillow.

SELECT BIBLIOGRAPHY
Cust 1902, p. 25; Venturi 1926, plate XLV; Larsen 1980a, p. 118, cat. 455; Barnes 1986, p. 381; T. Viscuso in Palermo 1990b, pp. 148–49, cat. I.4; Abbate 2001, pp. 87–88; Abbate 2004, pp. 70–71.

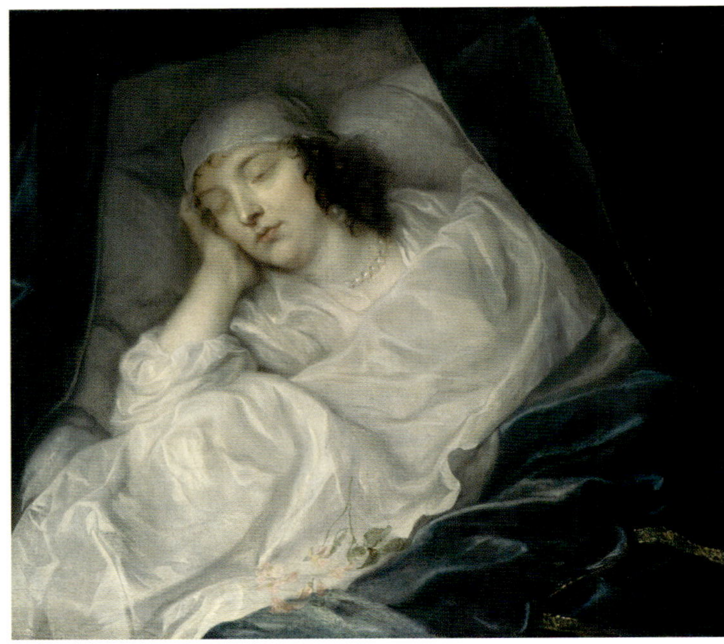

38 | Sir Anthony van Dyck, *Venetia Stanley, Lady Digby*
Dulwich Picture Gallery, London

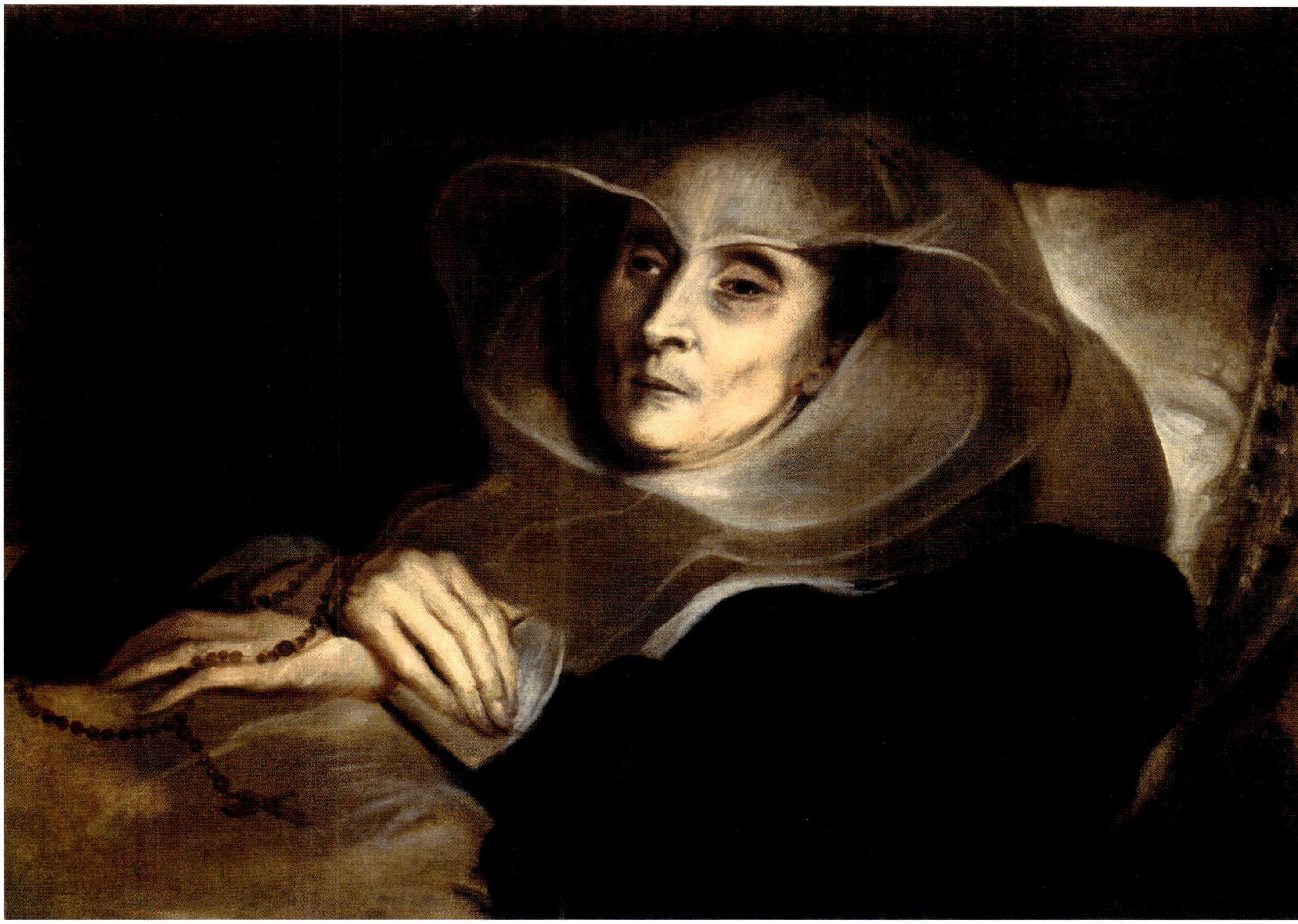

8 | Sir Anthony van Dyck

(1599–1641)

Desiderio Segno

1624
Oil on canvas, 131 × 101 cm
Inscribed on column at the right: AET.[S] 32. 1624
Liechtenstein.The Princely Collections, Vaduz-Vienna
(Inv. GE 61)

PROVENANCE

Desiderio Segno (d. 1630), Palermo and Salaparuta; probably acquired by Prince Johann Adam Andreas of Liechtenstein (1657–1712), Vienna, by 1733; part of Liechtenstein Collection, Vienna, until 1945; Liechtenstein Collection, Vaduz, until 2004; on display in the Liechtenstein Museum, Vienna.

Traditionally the painting has been recorded in the Liechtenstein Collection as a portrait of Albrecht Wenzel Eusebius von Wallenstein (1583–1634), the Bohemian general of the imperial troops in the Thirty Years' War. This identification has been subsequently questioned and Willem von Bode (1889) suggested that this may be a portrait of don Livio Odescalchi (1655–1713), nephew of Pope Innocent XI, even though the dates of the painter and the sitter do not match, as Van Dyck died almost fifteen years before Odescalchi's birth. The canvas is dated 1624 and the sitter is recorded as being thirty-two years old. As Van Dyck spent the first few months of 1624 in Genoa and most of the year in Palermo, it has been assumed that the sitter would be an Italian man; Larsen (1988) proposed that 'the sitter could conceivably be a nobleman from the court of Palermo'.

Vincenzo Abbate (1999b) persuasively related the Liechtenstein portrait with the documented portrait of Desiderio Segno. The painting appears in Segno's *post-mortem* inventory of 24 December 1630, a few days before he died, which lists 'a portrait of the deceased Signor Desiderio, by Anthony van Dyck, with a black frame' ('Un ritratto del quondam sign. Desiderio, di mano di Antonio Vandich, con guarnizione negra', Di Giovanni 1889, p. 287, see also Appendix 2). Segno also owned *Saint Rosalia in Glory Interceding for Palermo* (cat. 16), a *Deposition* and a 'head who yawns' by Van Dyck, together with other paintings by Luca Cambiaso and Sofonisba Anguissola. The date of birth of Desiderio Segno is unknown, but his father, Giovan Agostino, was born in 1566, so if Desiderio was thirty-two years old in 1624, it is possible that he was born in 1592, when his father was twenty-six. He was of the same generation as the Viceroy Emanuele Filiberto of Savoy, who was thirty-six in 1624. When Segno died in 1630 he left three young children, a boy and two girls, proving that he died at a relatively young age. He was of wealthy Genoese origins and ran his family's business together with his brother-in-law Giovan Agostino Arata. Between 1623 and 1624 he had been *console* of the Genoese community in Palermo, and was close to Orazio Lomellini, Sofonisba Anguissola's husband. It has even been suggested that Sofonisba may have been influential in shaping young Segno's artistic interests.

Apart from the portrait of the Viceroy Emanuele Filiberto of Savoy (cat. 2), and the images of Sofonisba Anguissola (cats. 5–6), no other portraits survive from Van Dyck's period in Sicily. The composition of the painting is strikingly similar to the portrait of the viceroy. Even though Desiderio Segno looks to the right and Emanuele Filiberto to the left, the body of the two sitters is positioned in an identical way. The sitters' left hands are very similar, in both cases limply resting on the hilt of the sword. It is possible that having seen the portrait of the viceroy in the summer of 1624, Segno commissioned his from Van Dyck. In contrast to the magnificent armour sported by Emanuele Filiberto, Segno is more simply and elegantly dressed. His black outfit is punctuated by crisp and refined white lace collar and cuffs. Behind him are a column and a chair that become props against which the image of the sitter is placed. Abbate suggested that the outfit, sword and the square diamond ring that Segno is wearing in the painting may be the same that appear in his inventory: 'trousers and jacket in black velvet [...] a sword [...] a gold ring with a diamond, broken in two' ('calzuni e gippone di velluto negro [...] una spata [...] un anello di oro, con uno diamante ingastato, rutto in dui pezzi'). However, the ring may be a fictional one, or an object that belonged to Van Dyck, as the exact same ring is also worn on the same finger of the left hand by Emanuele Filiberto in the Dulwich portrait.

Segno's features are handsomely rendered; the large blue watery eyes and the pallid skin contrast with the black clothes and dimly lit background. The fiery auburn hair, magnificent moustache and goatee characterise the striking features of the Genoese merchant, psychologically more human and vulnerable in comparison to Emanuele Filiberto's severe and haughty look. Abbate (1999b) proposed that Segno's right hand is meant to be interpreted as pointing towards something, as a sign ('segno' in Italian), in an intended allusion to the sitter's surname. The composition of the portrait is indebted to the example of Titian in particular. On his Italian travels, Van Dyck drew and recorded many of Titian's portraits in his *Sketchbook* (cat. 5), demonstrating his specific interest in the Venetian artist's approach to this genre of painting.

SELECT BIBLIOGRAPHY

Fanti 1767, vol. 1, cat. 257; Liechtenstein 1780, p. 220, cat. 670; Bode 1889, p. 49; Di Giovanni 1889, p. 287; Schaeffer 1909, p. 206; Glück 1931, p. 170; Van Puyvelde 1950, p. 113; Baldass 1957, p. 266; Larsen 1980a, p. 117, cat. 439; R. Baumstark in New York 1985, pp. 312–15, cat. 199; Barnes 1986, pp. 277–78, cat. 52; Larsen 1988, p. 151, cat. 372; Abbate 1999b, pp. 111–15; Abbate 2004, pp. 72, 75–76; S.J. Barnes in Barnes, De Poorter, Millar, Vey 2004, pp. 202–03, cat. II.61; A. Merle du Bourg in Paris 2008, pp. 68–69, cat. 10; Abbate 2011, pp. 90–94.

EXHIBITIONS

Meisterwerke aus den Sammlungen des Fürsten von Liechtenstein, Kunstmuseum, Lucerne 1948, cat. 121; *Liechtenstein: The Princely Collections*, The Metropolitan Museum of Art, New York, 1985–86, cat. 199; *Antoon van Dyck. Portraits*, Musée Jacquemart-André, Paris 2008–09, cat. 10.

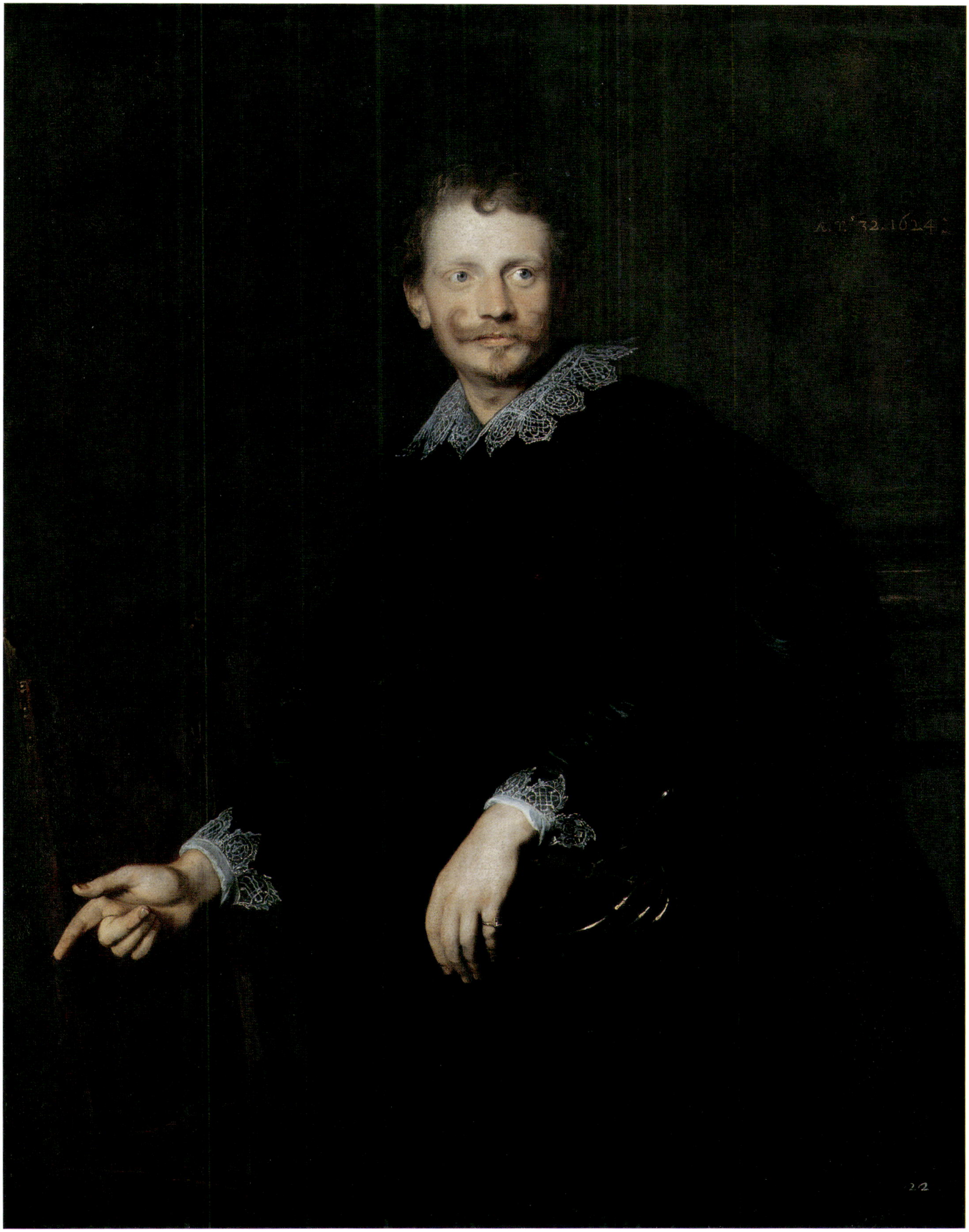

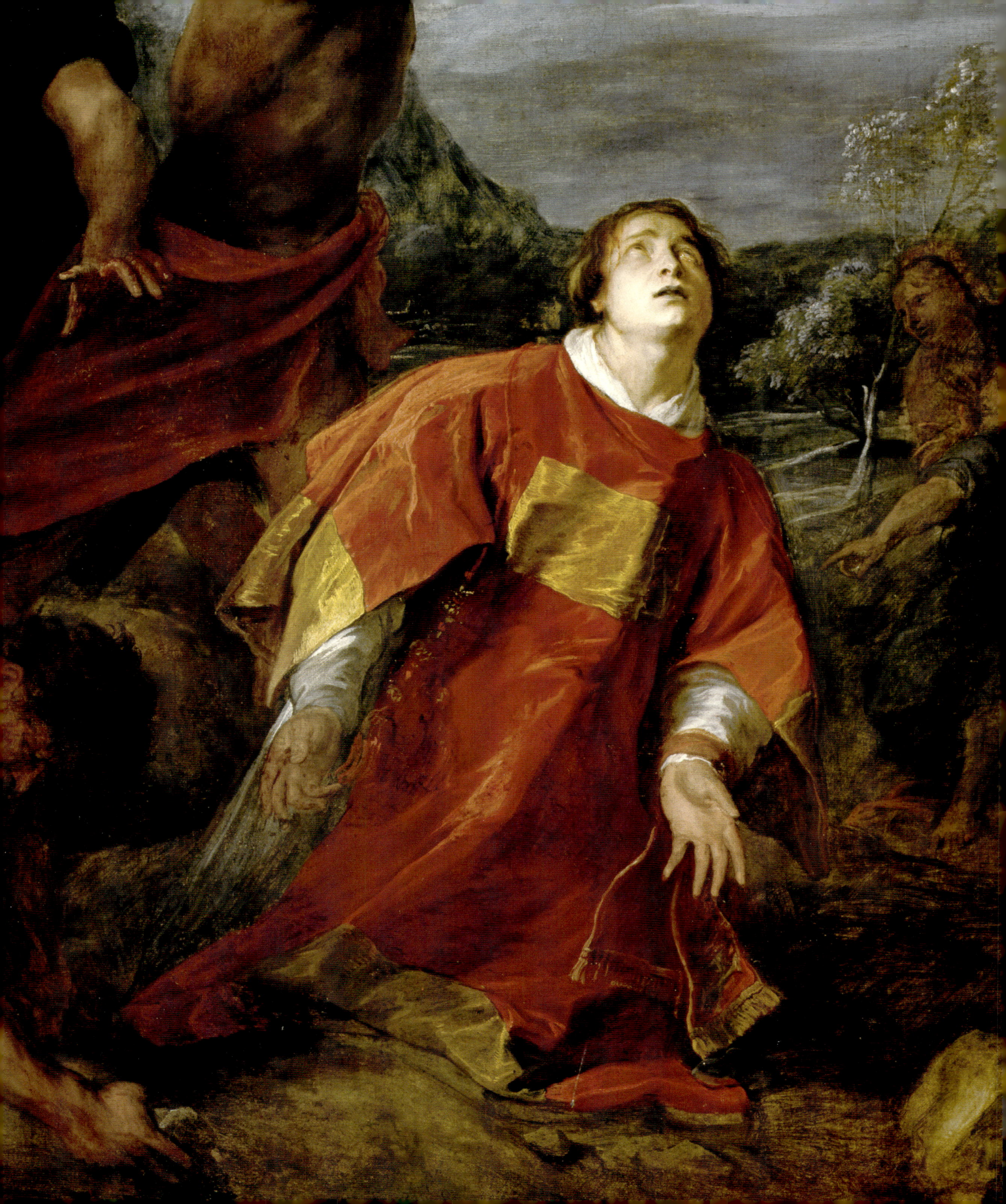

Devotional Paintings

9 | Sir Anthony van Dyck
(1599–1641)

Stoning of Saint Stephen

c. 1624
Oil on canvas, 178 × 150 cm
Tatton Park, The Egerton Collection (The National Trust)
(Inv. TAT/P/39)

PROVENANCE
Possibly painted for Fabrizio Valguarnera (d. 1632), Palermo, and brought to Madrid in 1628; San Pascual Bailon, Madrid, 1776; Manuel de Godoy (1767–1851), Principe de la Paz, from between 1803 and 1806; George Augustus Wallis (1761–1847), acting for William Buchanan (1777–1864), 1808; brought to England in 1813; Alexis Delahante (1767–1837); his sale, Phillips, London, 3 June 1814 (lot 77); bought Wilbraham Egerton of Tatton (1781–1856); by descent to the Barons Egerton of Tatton, Tatton Park; left with Tatton Park to the National Trust in 1958 by Maurice, 4th and last Baron Egerton of Tatton (1874–1958).

According to the Acts of the Apostles, in the early days of the Christian Church, after the resurrection and ascension of Christ, the apostles recruited seven deacons and among them Stephen, a man 'full of faith and power', who 'did great wonders and miracles among the people' (Acts 6:8). Stephen was the first martyr of Christianity; captured by the people he was preaching to, 'then they cried out with a loud voice, and stopped their ears, and ran upon him with one accord, and cast him out of the city, and stoned him: and the witnesses laid down their clothes at a young man's feet, whose name was Saul. And they stoned Stephen, calling upon God, and saying, Lord Jesus, receive my spirit. And he kneeled down, and cried with a loud voice, Lord, lay not this sin to their charge. And when he had said this, he fell asleep' (Acts 7:57–60).

Van Dyck set the scene in a wide landscape, with trees rustling in stormy winds. The sky is dramatically clouded, as it darkens around the martyr's final moments. Five men lift stones and violently throw them on Stephen; behind them an onlooker witnesses the scene. The saint kneels, dressed in a bright red and gold dalmatic, and gazes to heaven. He has already been hit by stones and is wounded in the head; blood is coming out of his nose and his eyes are filled with tears. Stephen's last moments are vividly captured, as his already livid lips utter his last words of forgiveness. The figure in the right background is Saul (the future Saint Paul), as described by the Acts, with the clothes of the witnesses at his feet. From heaven two angels descend with a palm branch and martyr's crowns for Stephen. In composition, the painting is particularly close to Rubens's altarpiece of the *Stoning of Saint Stephen*, painted around 1615–20, when Van Dyck was in his workshop, and now in the Musée des Beaux-Arts in Valenciennes. Van Dyck also looked at other sources such as Raphael's Vatican tapestry of the same subject, and Titian's altarpiece of *Saint Peter Martyr* in SS. Giovanni e Paolo in Venice. In Genoa, Van Dyck must also have studied carefully Giulio Romano's and Giovan Battista Paggi's two altarpieces, both of which also depicted the *Stoning of Saint Stephen* in the churches of Santo Stefano and the Gesù.

Antonio Ponz in his *Viage de España* (1776) described on the altar of the fourth chapel to the left in the church of San Pascual Bailon in Madrid 'the martyrdom of Saint Sebastian, painted by Anthony van Dyck' ('En el altar de la quarta Capilla se vé el martirio de S. Esteban, pintado por Antonio Van-Dik'). It has been proposed that, together with other paintings in the church – possibly including Van Dyck's *Saint Rosalia* in Houston (cat. 14) – the canvas was donated to the church by don Juan Gaspar Enríquez de Cabrera, 6th Duque de Medina de Rosecí and 10th Almirante de Castilla (1623–91), whose father may have acquired it in Italy. Between 1803 and 1806 the *Stoning of Saint Stephen* was removed from the church by don Manuel Godoy, who displayed it in his palace in Madrid until his fall from power and arrest in 1808. The English artist George Augustus Wallis bought the painting in that year, on behalf of the dealer William Buchanan, and brought it to England in 1813, passing through Germany and France. Having acquired the canvas for more than 1,000 pounds, the dealer Alexis Delahante sold the picture on 3 June 1814 for 700 guineas (735 pounds) to Wilbraham Egerton of Tatton, through whose descendants the canvas remained at Tatton Park.

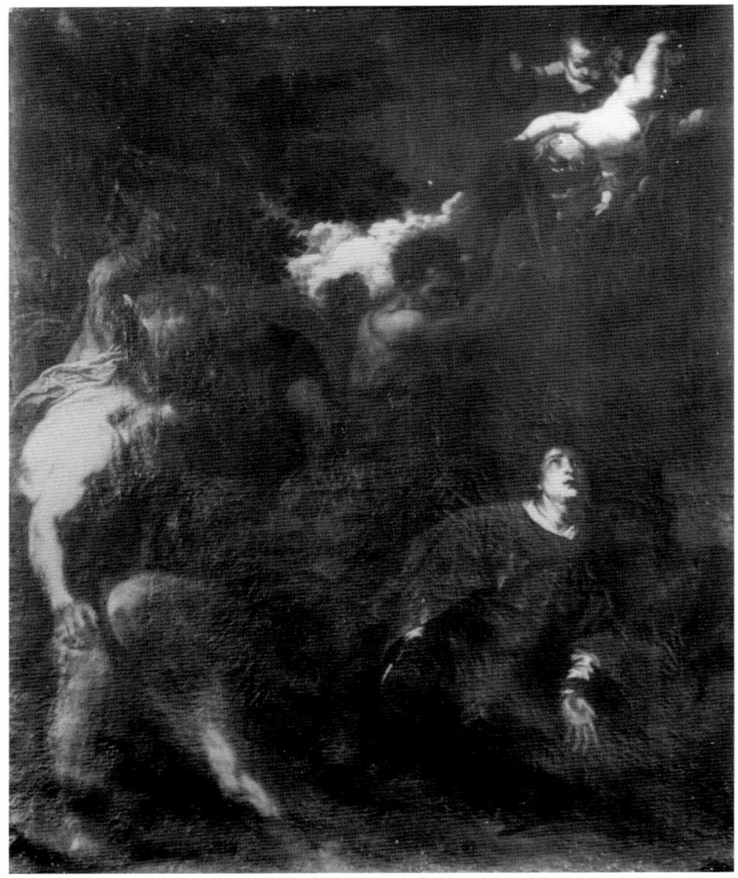
39 | After Sir Anthony van Dyck, *Stoning of Saint Stephen*, Private Collection, Palermo

The original commission of the painting is unknown. The catalogue of Delahante's sale in 1814 recorded that the *Stoning of Saint Stephen* was 'painted at Venice by the immortal artist, for the Spanish chapel at Rome' and since then a possible provenance from San Giacomo degli Spagnoli in Rome has generally been accepted (Cust 1900 first men-

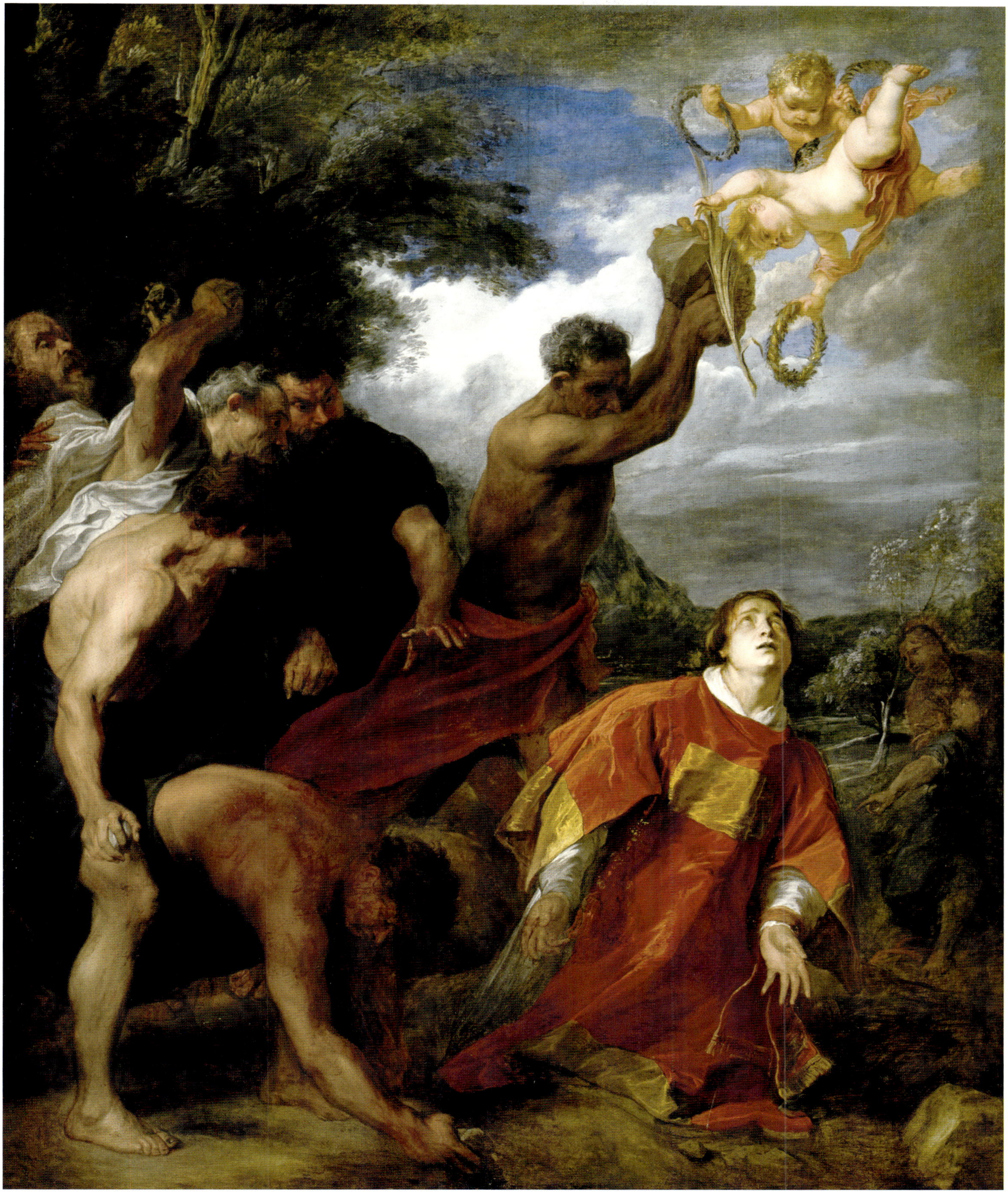

tioned this specific church). However, it is highly unlikely that if Van Dyck painted a public altarpiece for a church in Rome during his Italian sojourn it would have been altogether unrecorded, especially in Bellori's biography. The statement in the catalogue is most likely to be incorrect. Stylistically the picture is placed during Van Dyck's Italian period, between 1621 and 1627. Christopher Brown (1995b and 1999a) has rightly noticed the similarity between the head of Saint Stephen and the two angels in the Tatton Park painting with the head of the saint and angels in the series of images of Saint Rosalia that Van Dyck painted in Palermo (cats. 12–16), and suggested a more specific date of around 1623–25. Susan Barnes (2004) wrote that 'the Spanish provenance could point to the painting's having been in Sicily'. The existence of two copies of the painting, in a private collection in Palermo (now untraced – fig. 39) and in the Castello Ursino in Catania, supports Barnes's claim (Abbate 2004, p. 77 n. 38). Barnes also noticed that 'although the size and subject are appropriate for an altarpiece, it might instead have been made for the open market, or for a private collector in any of the Italian cities in which Van Dyck worked'.

On 22 April 1626 Desiderio Segno (cat. 8) signed a document in which he claimed that he was holding a group of paintings as security against 80 *onze* he had lent to Fabrizio Valguarnera on 6 May 1624. Four of these paintings were said to be by Titian; the fifth was a '*Martyrdom of Saint Stephen* said to be by the hand of Anthony van Dyck' ('nec non un quatro del martirio di Santo Stefano quod dicunt che sia di mano di Antonio Vandich fiamengo di altezza di nove palmi incirca, e sette palmi incirca di larghezza'; Mendola 1999c, p. 61). Giovanni Mendola (1999c), publishing this piece of information, linked this document to the Tatton Park painting and suggested that its copy in a private collection in Palermo (fig. 39) may have been Valguarnera's picture. The *Stoning of Saint Stephen* belonging to Valguarnera measured – according to the 1626 document – 9 × 7 *palmi*, corresponding to 225 × 175 cm and would have been slightly larger than the Tatton Park painting. Vincenzo Abbate (2004) also connected Valguarnera's canvas with the Palermo copy, but tentatively suggested that instead the Tatton Park picture could have been Valguarnera's and may have been cut down. In fact the identification of Valguarnera's *Saint Stephen* with the Tatton Park painting seems to be logical. If the painting was not cut down, the compiler of the 1626 document may have reported the framed dimensions of the canvas. It is well known that Valguarnera owned original canvases by celebrated artists and he also often commissioned and owned copies after them, possibly intended for nefarious market purposes. He commissioned Hieronymus Gerards's copies of his four Old Testament scenes by Titian, and had Angelo Caroselli copy Nicolas Poussin's *Plague at Ashdod*, which he also owned. Furthermore, the documents of Valguarnera's trial in Rome in 1631 state that when he travelled from Palermo to Madrid in 1628, he brought his collection of paintings with him and sold them there (Costello 1950, p. 260). This could explain how the *Stoning of Saint Stephen* reached Spain; its copies, instead, must have remained in Sicily.

Valguarnera's commission of the painting must have been dictated by a particular veneration for Saint Stephen. In his will, of 25 December 1631, Valguarnera invoked 'the most Holy Trinity, Father, Son, and Holy Ghost, the Immaculate Virgin Mary, the sinners' intercessor, Saint Michael Archangel, Saint Stephen, Saint Anthony of Padua, and my other protectors and intercessors of the entire celestial hierarchy' ('in nome della S.ma Trinità, Padre, Figliolo, e Spirito Santo, et dell'Immacolata Vergine Maria Avocata de' Peccatori, di S. Michel Arcangelo, S. Stefano, S. Antonio di Padua, et altri miei Protettori, et Avocati di tutta la celeste Gerarchia'; Rome 1994, p. 233). The head of the figure on the extreme left of the painting, witnessing Stephen's martyrdom, but not taking part in it, is particularly individualised and it is likely to be a specific portrait. This has not been noticed before, even though it is not unusual for donor portraits to appear in religious narratives. The trial documents describe in detail Valguarnera's appearance when he appeared in court on 13 July 1631: 'of medium height, aged about thirty-eight, black hair, of a reddish complexion, chestnut beard, with long moustaches, face rather full… dressed in the following clothing, that is, in a hat of black felt with cords, cloak… of black Spanish silk and wool, stockings of black silk, shoes of black chamois with knotted black ribbons, in sleeves of black watered taffeta, in a bodice of damask of turquoise blue trimmed with silver lace, in breeches of black watered taffeta' (Costello 1950, p. 257). The man in the Tatton Park picture corresponds to most of these details, especially with his full face, reddish complexion, and chestnut beard with full moustache. It is probable that this may be the only surviving portrait of Fabrizio Valguarnera.

SELECT BIBLIOGRAPHY

Ponz 1776, vol. 5, p. 38; Buchanan 1824, vol. 2, pp. 238–41, 245, 247; Smith 1831, vol. 3, p. 100, cat. 354; Guiffrey 1882, p. 55; Cust 1900, p. 240, cat. 48; London 1900, p. 36, cat. 89; Glück 1931, p. 137; Du Gué Trapier 1957, p. 269; Gaya Nuño 1964, pp. 44–45; J.R. Martin and G. Feigenbaum in Princeton 1979, pp. 24–25; Larsen 1980a, p. 114, cat. 407; Brigstocke 1982, p. 18; Rose 1983, vol. 2, pp. 121–23; Barnes 1986, pp. 176–79, cat. 15; Larsen 1988, p. 190, cat. 471; Abbate 1990, pp. 46–47; C. Brown in London 1995b, pp. 132–33, cat. 49; Abbate 1999b, p. 131 n. 42; C. Brown in London 1999a, pp. 166–67, cat. 32; Mendola 1999b, p. 101; Mendola 1999c, p. 62; Abbate 2004, pp. 73, 76–77; S.J. Barnes in Barnes, De Poorter, Millar, Vey 2004, pp. 164–65, cat. II.19.

EXHIBITIONS

Winter Exhibition, Royal Academy of Arts, London 1884, cat. 166; *Exhibition of the Works by Van Dyck 1599–1641*, Royal Academy of Arts, London 1900, cat. 89; *Italian Art*, Royal Academy of Arts, London 1960, cat. 51; *Van Dyck*, Agnew's, London 1968, cat. 19; *In Trust for the Nation. Paintings from National Trust Houses*, The National Gallery, London 1995, cat. 49; *Van Dyck 1599–1641*, Koninklijk Museum voor Schone Kunsten, Antwerp, and Royal Academy of Arts, London 1999, cat. 32.

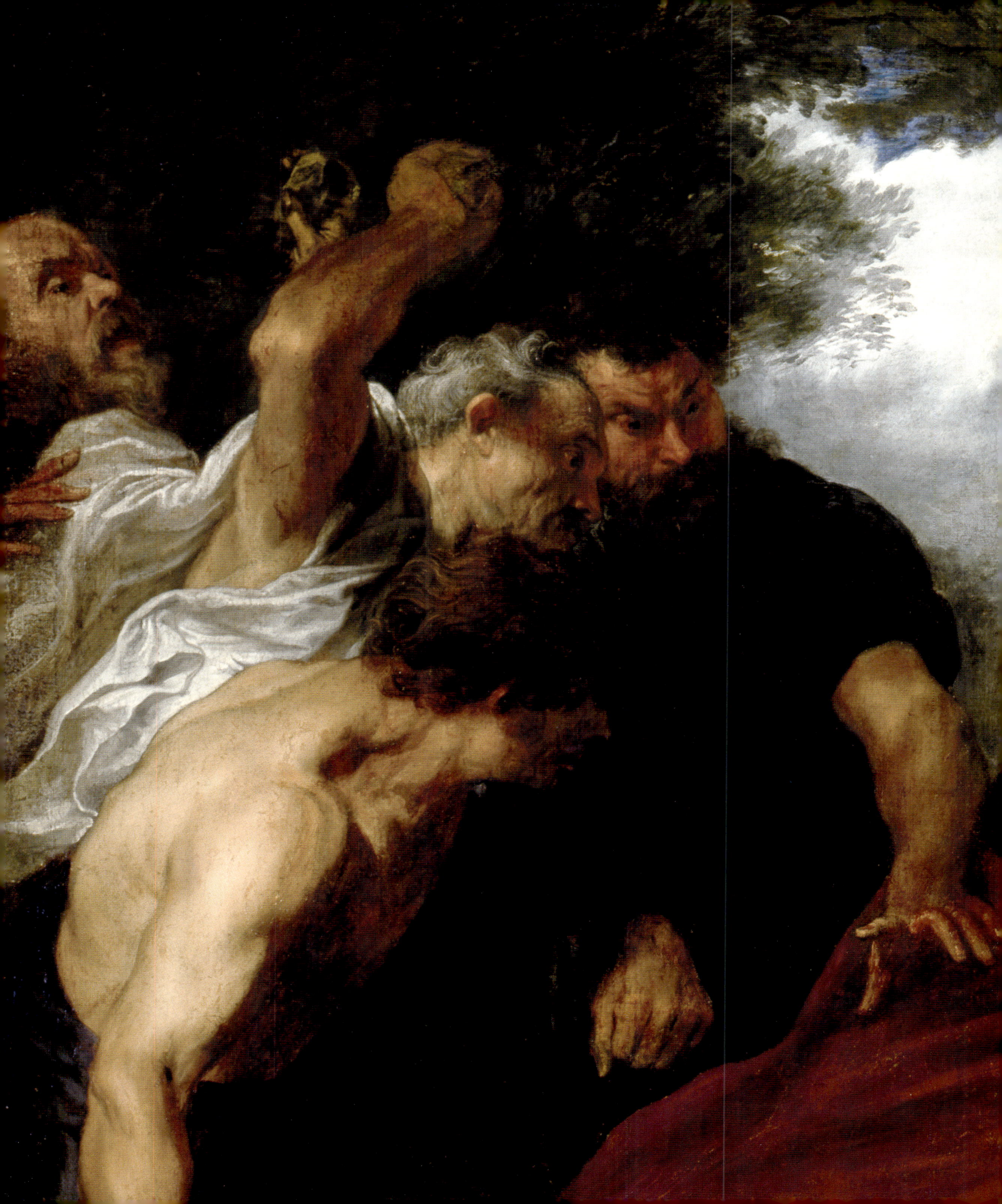

10 | Sir Anthony van Dyck
(1599–1641)

Saint John the Baptist in the Wilderness

c. 1624–25
Oil on canvas, 141 × 115 cm
Houston Baptist University, Houston
Gift of the Morris Collection, 2009

PROVENANCE

Possibly Spanish Royal Collection, Buen Retiro Palace, Madrid; possibly Jean-Gilbert-Victor Fialin, Duc de Persigny (1808–72); Maurice Cottier, Paris; Daniel Cottier, Cottier & Co., New York and London; Walter P. Fearon, New York, by 1925; Stephen S. Picchetto, New York, by 1939; Central Picture Galleries, by 1979; Los Angeles County Museum of Art, 1994; Christie's, New York, 26 January 2001 (lot 82); William and Sharon Morris, Houston; their gift to Houston Baptist University, 2009.

The large painting of *Saint John the Baptist* is close in style to other religious paintings by Van Dyck from his Italian period, in particular the *Martyrdom of Saint Sebastian* in the Alte Pinakothek in Munich (S.J. Barnes in Barnes, De Poorter, Millar, Vey 2004, pp. 163–64, cat. II.18). Susan Barnes (1986) originally rejected the attribution to the painter, but later revised her opinion suggesting that the canvas was painted around 1621–22, as soon as Van Dyck arrived in Genoa. Oliver Millar (1997), instead, partly questioning the attribution, placed the painting during Van Dyck's second Genoese period or early after his return to Flanders, in 1627. Even though it is usually said that this work is documented in the Spanish Royal Collection in the palace of the Buen Retiro in Madrid, between 1700 and 1808, there is no evidence for such assertion, as demonstrated by Martin and Feigenbaum (1979). Glück (1931) tentatively connected this work to Bellori's reference to a 'Saint John the Baptist in the wilderness' ('San Gio. Battista nel deserto' – Bellori 2005, p. 219; Bellori 2009, p. 281) painted for Sir Kenelm Digby and dated it to 1623–25. It is clear, however, that the picture described by Bellori was made in England, and the painting in Houston has all the stylistic traits of an Italian work by Van Dyck. Even the canvas used for the *Saint John the Baptist* is a diamond-pattern table cloth, often employed by southern Italian artists in the seventeenth century.

Saint John the Baptist is depicted full-length, sitting at the entrance to a cave (like Saint Rosalia in Van Dyck's paintings). Behind him on the right there is a landscape with a view over a valley with woods and a tower. The saint is nude and wears only a voluminous scarlet robe that barely covers him. He reads from a book that he holds in his left hand, and with his right he grips a wooden cross, around which a white banner is intertwined, with the inscription: 'Ecce Agnus Dei, qui tollit peccatum mundi' (John 1:29). At his feet, half hidden in shadow, is his traditional attribute of the lamb.

The influence of artists such as Guido Reni and Massimo Stanzione on Van Dyck has been mentioned in connection to this canvas. The composition is powerfully Caravaggesque and it is not unlikely that the Flemish painter knew Caravaggio's *Saint John the Baptist* (Nelson Atkins Museum of Art, Kansas City) painted for the Genoese banker Ottavio Costa. He may have seen the original in Rome, or possibly the contemporary copy that the Costa family had in their castle at Conscente, near Genoa.

Giovanni Mendola (1999c), considering the influence of this work on Sicilian artists such as Pietro Novelli, reasonably proposed that Van Dyck may have painted the *Saint John the Baptist* in Palermo in 1624–25. This may indeed be identified, as argued by Mendola, with the 'large painting of Saint John' ('un quatro grande di San gio: di mano di ant vandic con taffita del proprio modo') listed in the inventory of Simone Sitaiolo on 20 March 1632.

SELECT BIBLIOGRAPHY

Glück 1925, pp. 26–31; Glück 1931, pp. XXXVI, 138; J.R. Martin and G. Feigenbaum in Princeton 1979, pp. 120–21, cat. 32; Larsen 1980a, p. 116, cat. 433; Barnes 1986, p. 380; Little 1995; S.J. Barnes in Genoa 1997, pp. 322–23, cat. 68; Millar 1997, p. 502; Stewart 1997, p. 53; Mendola 1999c, p. 62; S.J. Barnes in Barnes, De Poorter, Millar, Vey 2004, p. 159, cat. II.13.

EXHIBITIONS

Loan Exhibition of Dutch Paintings of the Seventeenth Century, Detroit Institute of Arts, Detroit 1925, cat. 31; *Fifty Paintings by Van Dyck*, Detroit Institute of Arts, Detroit 1929, cat. 18; *Masterpieces of Art*, New York World's Fair, New York 1939, cat. 101; *Van Dyck as Religious Artist*, The Art Museum, Princeton University, Princeton, New Jersey 1979, cat. 32; *Van Dyck a Genova. Grande pittura e collezionismo*, Palazzo Ducale, Genoa 1997, cat. 68.

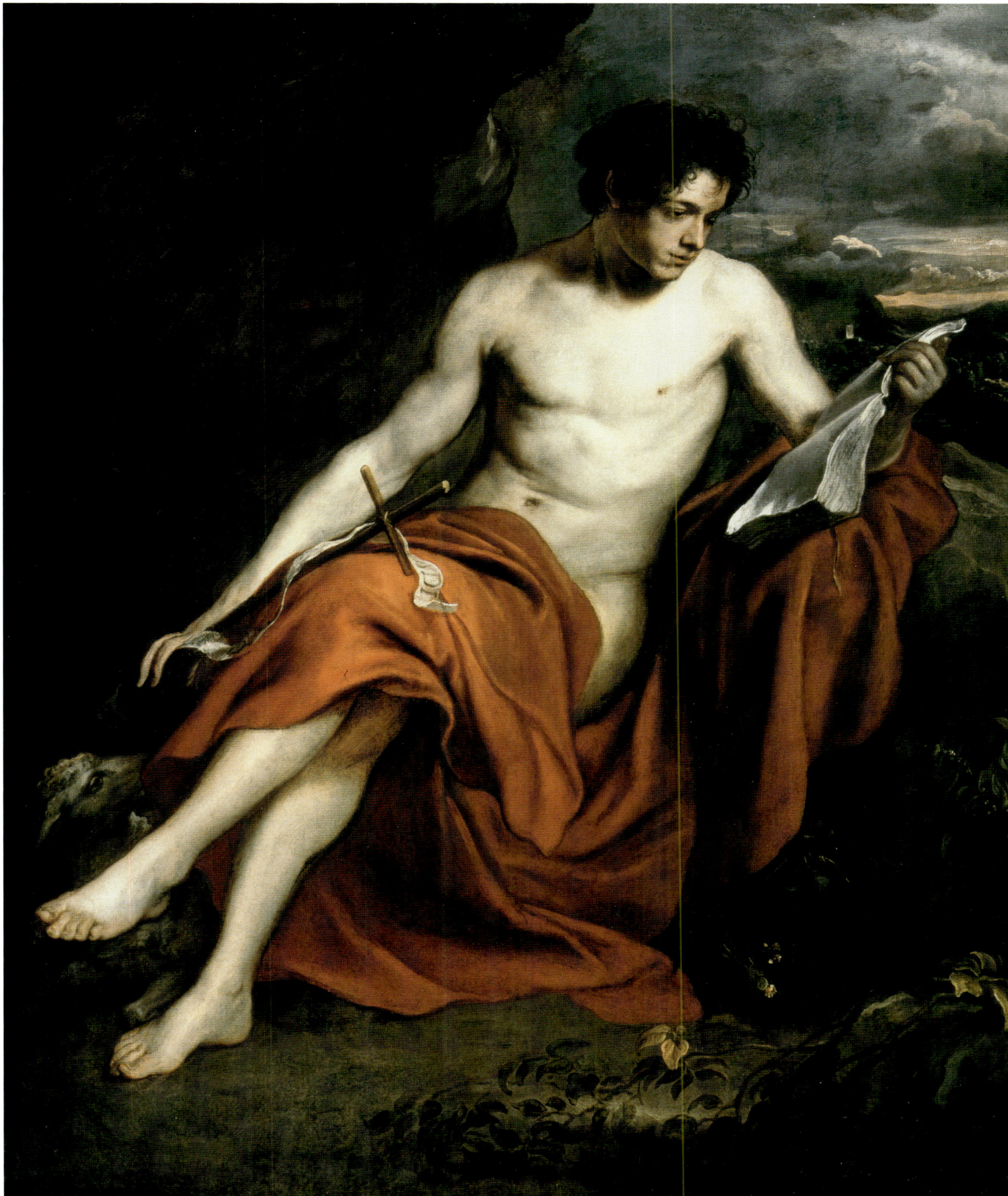

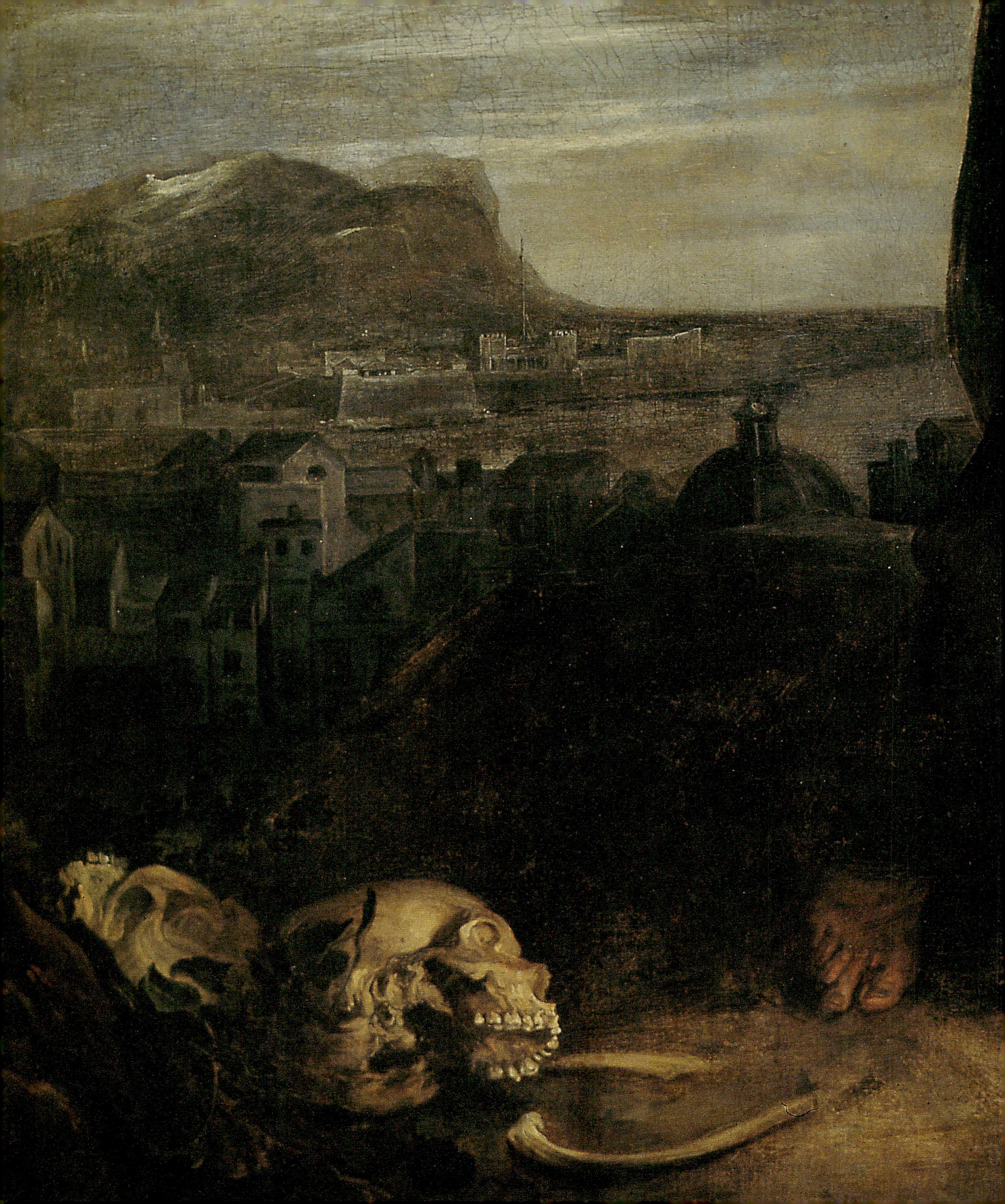

Saint Rosalia

11 | Vincenzo La Barbera

(*c.* 1577–*c.* 1653)

Saint Rosalia Interceding for Palermo

1624
Oil on canvas, 154.5 × 103.5 cm
Museo Diocesano, Palermo
(Inv. 484)

PROVENANCE

Probably commissioned by the Senate of Palermo on 27 July 1624; Cathedral of Palermo; deposited from Archivio Storico Comunale to Municipio of Palermo, 1904; Museo Diocesano, Palermo.

This is likely to be the image of Saint Rosalia commissioned by the Senate of Palermo from Vincenzo La Barbera on 27 July 1624 for the fee of 67 *onze* and 6 *tarì* (Collura 1977, p. 77). The painting was ready on 24 August and, on 4 September of that year, it was brought in a solemn procession around the city as a remedy against the plague. On 14 September La Barbera was paid 50 *onze* by the Senate 'for having painted a new picture of the image of Saint Rosalia' ('pro magisterio unius quatri noviter facti immaginae S. Rosaliae'). It is unclear if the canvas was ultimately intended for a specific location, but this is the first documented portrayal of the saint in the wake of the discovery of her relics during the plague of 1624.

Vincenzo La Barbera (for whom, see Contino and Mantia 1998) was born in Termini Imerese, east of Palermo, around 1577, from a family of Genoese origins. He was an architect and painter and as a young man trained in Termini with Antonino Spatafora. In 1597 he married Spatafora's daughter Elisabetta. From June 1613 La Barbera is recorded as 'capomastro delle fabbriche della città di Termini'. He must have been a successful painter, and his works were produced for many Sicilian towns, including Caccamo, Ciminna, Vicari, Montemaggiore, Polizzi, Collesano and Mussomeli. In 1622 he moved to Palermo where, in that year, he designed the decorations for the canonisation of Saint Ignatius of Loyola and Saint Francis Xavier. He was closely connected to the Jesuits and designed the marble decoration of the Jesuit church in Palermo, known as Casa Professa. He also provided designs for *palliotti* for altars and tapestries. For the first *festino* of Saint Rosalia in 1625 he designed with Pietro Alvino the triumphal arches for the Senate and for the Genoese community. He died around 1653. La Barbera is likely to have been particularly devoted to Saint Rosalia. His daughter was said to have been miraculously cured from the plague through the saint's intercession, and his son, Francesco – who later became a priest and architect – uttered, only eighteen months old, the name of Rosalia and knelt upon seeing for the first time the small relics of the saint that his father owned (Giordano 1997, pp. 277–82; Collura 1977, p. 96).

Saint Rosalia is depicted, full-length, interceding for the city of Palermo during the plague. She is shown with a halo, in a brown monastic dress, set against the background of the city of Palermo. Above the saint, over a cloud and surrounded by a glory of angels, are the Holy Trinity and the Virgin Mary. On the ground, next to Rosalia, is a book surmounted by a skull, next to a lily. The saint looks up to the celestial vision, while a small angel brings her a crown of roses. The key elements of the iconography of Saint Rosalia are established here: the dress, skull, book, lily and crown of roses. These provided the basis on which Van Dyck constructed his representations of Rosalia. In the background La Barbera depicted an accurate view of Palermo in 1624, and in particular of the area where Van Dyck lived, next to the harbour. Rosalia points to the Lazzaretto, the hospital for the plague's victims, and to the right La Cala (the harbour) can be seen, from Porta Felice, the Castello a Mare and the Monte Pellegrino in the background, just below the Trinity.

The upper section of the painting seems of poorer quality than the lower part, and it has convincingly been given to La Barbera's workshop (Abbate 1991, p. 99). A year later La Barbera produced another painting of Saint Rosalia, now in the church of Sant'Anna la Misericordia (fig. 27). This was commissioned from the artist on 25 February 1625 by the lawyer Andrea La Barbera e Restivo for his burial chapel in Sant'Anna (ASP, Not. Pietro Levantino, vol. 15837, f. 269; Mendola 1999a, pp. 65–66). La Barbera was asked by the patron to produce a *modello* of the painting ('sguaczo di cartollone') before the altarpiece could be approved. In this second painting the composition is on the whole comparable with the one of the canvas in the Museo Diocesano. The view of Palermo during the plague, however, is made even more dramatic by the addition of a pile of corpses next to Rosalia, which the saint points towards while looking up to the Trinity and the Virgin.

SELECT BIBLIOGRAPHY

Collura 1977, p. 96; Abbate 1991, pp. 99–101; Di Natale 1998, p. 92; A. Cuccia in Palermo 1999, p. 274; Palazzotto 2003, pp. 8–11, 29; Bailey 2005, pp. 124–25; Di Natale 2006, pp. 90, 96–98.

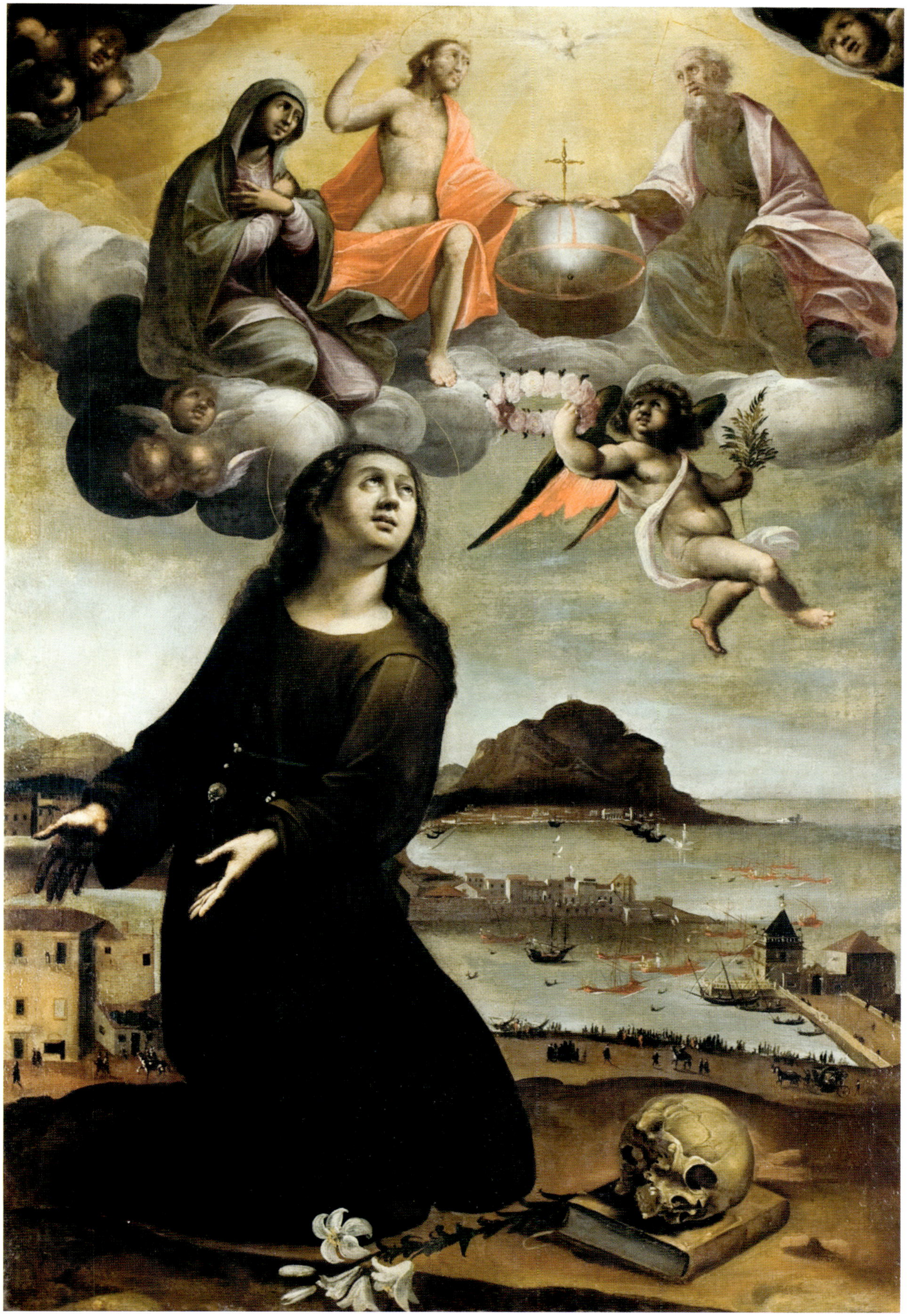

12 | Sir Anthony van Dyck
(1599–1641)

Saint Rosalia Interceding for Palermo

c. 1624–25
Oil on canvas, 172.1 × 146.1 cm
Museo de Arte de Ponce, The Luis A. Ferré Foundation Inc., Ponce, Puerto Rico
(Inv. 60.0159)

PROVENANCE
Said to be a gift from Louis II de Bourbon, Prince de Condé (1621–86) to the Marquis de Cossart d'Espiès, Château d'Omécourt; Baron de Coriolis, Paris, by 1939; Sotheby's, London, 7 December 1960 (lot 122); acquired by Luis A. Ferré for Museo de Arte de Ponce.

When first published by Charles Sterling in 1939 the painting belonged to the Baron de Coriolis in Paris. A forged Murillo signature had been added to the canvas as it was displayed as a pendant to a copy of Murillo's *Two Boys* at Dulwich Picture Gallery, in the Château d'Omécourt in the Beauvaisie (Sterling 1939, p. 59 n. 25). The Château was the seat of the Cossart d'Espiès family, and the picture was traditionally said to have been a gift from Louis II de Bourbon, the Grand Condé, to the Marquis de Cossart d'Espiès. From the French Revolution onwards the canvas appeared in inventories of the Cossart family.

Sterling (1939, p. 60) noted that 'the picture is thin and smooth in surface. This can partly be accounted for by the cleaning and backing to which it was submitted in the past and which have worn away and flattened down the paint', but he also proposed that the canvas on which it was painted was of Northern facture. He, therefore, dated the painting to 1629, arguing that it was produced by Van Dyck in Antwerp, after he returned from Italy. He concluded that 'the actual face of the saint, tender and rounded, is akin to the faces of the Antwerp period and wholly different from the firmer, more ardent, Titianesque type of the Ospedale dei Sacerdoti copy'. Sterling stressed in general the difference between this picture and the *Saint Rosalia* in Houston (cat. 14), which he placed during the Italian period. In general, this view has been followed until the present (Gordon 1979; Barnes 1986; Vey 2004 commented that 'the application of paint is thin and smooth, in contrast to the Italian paintings, the colours are cooler and the forms firmer; additionally, the facial type is Northern'; Hale 2008). However, as convincingly argued by Bailey (2005), it is more likely that the painting was produced in Palermo in 1624–25 and that this, being almost identical in composition to Vincenzo La Barbera's *Saint Rosalia Interceding for Palermo*, commissioned by the Senate of the city in July 1624 (cat. 11), was the first image of Saint Rosalia produced by Van Dyck in Sicily. It is impossible to establish if this painting is the *Saint Rosalia* that appears in the inventory of 20 March 1632 of Simone Sitaiolo (Mendola 1999b, p. 101; Mendola 1999c, p. 61; Abbate 2004, p. 74), but it cannot be identified with the other picture of the same subject that is recorded in the 1658 inventory of Marco Gezio (Morreale 1990, p. 44; Mendola 1999b, p. 101; Mendola 1999c, p. 61; Abbate 2004, p. 77) – the size of this last painting is documented as being 5 × 4 *palmi* (approximately 129 × 103 cm), much smaller than the Ponce canvas.

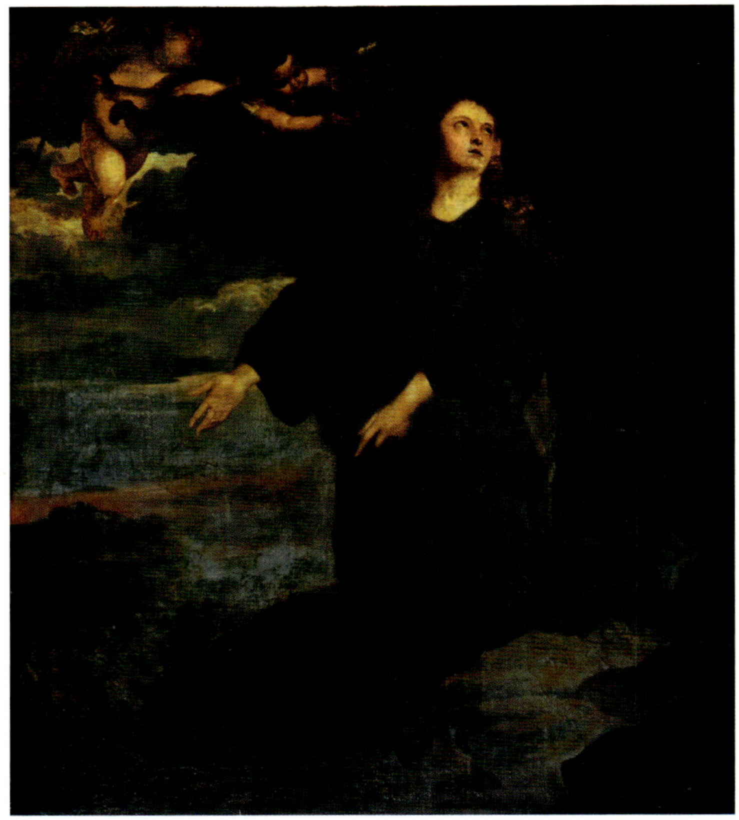

40 | After Sir Anthony van Dyck, *Saint Rosalia Interceding for Palermo*
Cappella dei Santi Pietro e Paolo dell'Infermeria dei Sacerdoti, Palermo

Saint Rosalia appears kneeling outside her cave, pointing below to the city of Palermo. In her pose the figure exactly matches the one in La Barbera's painting. She gazes upwards, as her hands point to the city she is interceding for. The celestial vision in La Barbera's painting has been eliminated and replaced by divine light that descends from the top right corner. Rosalia has been shifted to the right side of the picture, and below her are a skull and bones. She is wearing a simple grey monastic dress, with a transparent veil; her auburn hair is loose over her shoulders. Behind her, at the mouth of the cave, is a rolled woven straw mat, which the saint used as a bed. To the left the cave looks out onto a landscape of Palermo, less precise than La Barbera's but geographically similar. From her cave, located on the Monte Pellegrino, the saint points to a depiction of the same location; the Monte Pellegrino itself appears in the background behind Palermo. Sterling (1939, p. 62) argued that 'the view of the town… shows that the original work was intended for Palermo, probably at the moment of the city's tragic passion' and identifies the view as taken from the Palazzo dei Normanni, with the dome of the Cathedral next to the saint. The area represented in the painting, however, like in La Barbera's canvas, is that of La Cala, on the opposite side of the city from the Cathedral and Palazzo dei Normanni. This is the zone near the churches of Santa Maria di Portosalvo and Santa Maria della Catena, where Van Dyck lived as a guest of the Flemish consul, Hendrik Dych.

A copy of the painting survives in Palermo, in the Cappella dei Santi Pietro e Paolo dell'Infermeria dei

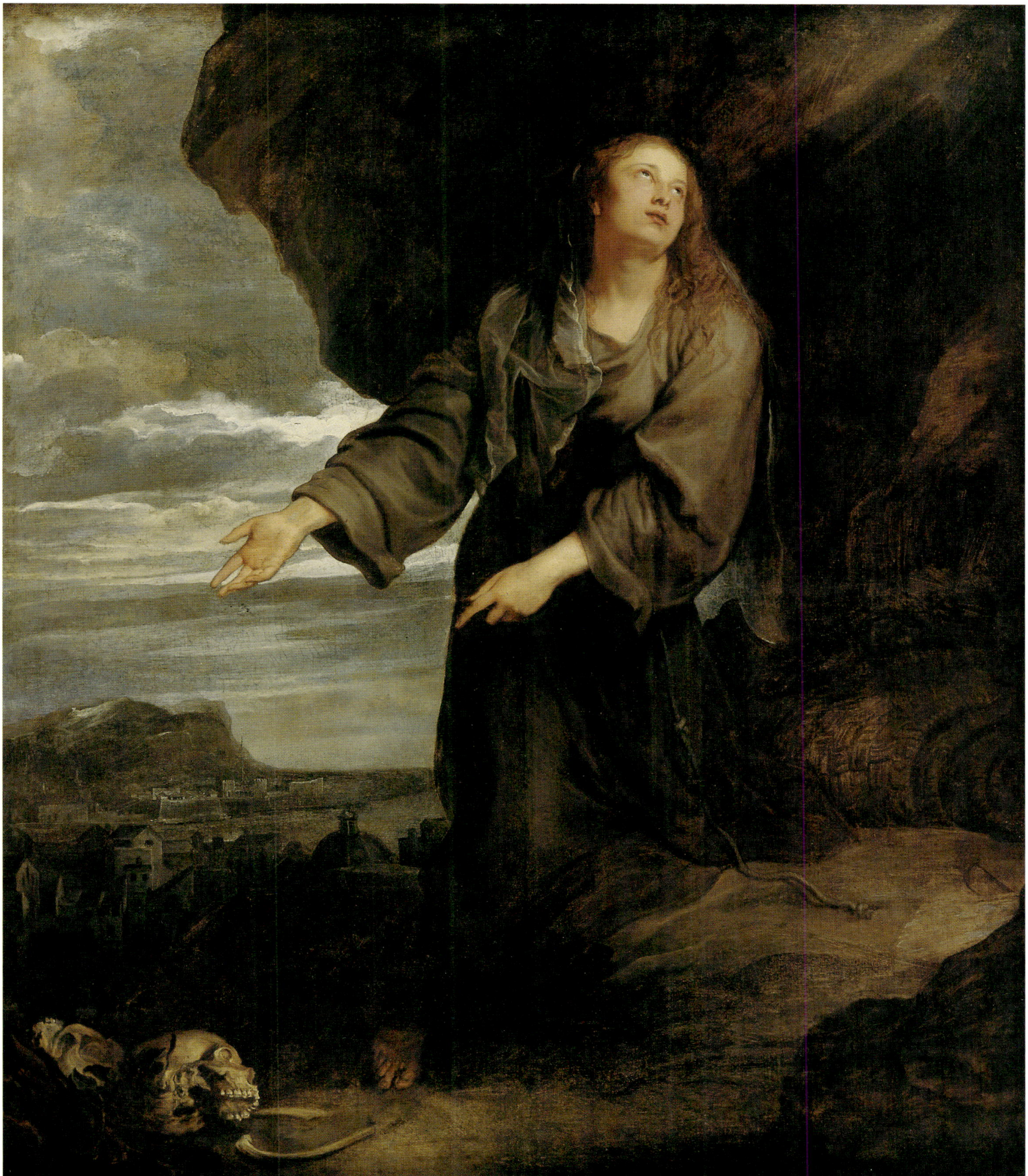

Sacerdoti (also known as the Ospedale dei Sacerdoti – fig. 40). Cesare Matranga (1908, p. 15) hypothesises that the copy after Van Dyck's work was brought from Spain by the founder of the Ospedale dei Sacerdoti, the Archbishop don Fernando de Bazán, who instituted the chapel in 1698. However, there is no documentary evidence that the copy reached Palermo from Spain, and it is more likely that both original and copy were painted in Palermo. The canvas in the Ospedale dei Sacerdoti is identical to the Ponce painting, with the exception of the two angels at the top left, crowning Saint Rosalia. They are very close in style to Van Dyck's work and it is unclear if they record a detail that was in the original and was subsequently covered up (no X-ray image of the Ponce painting has been taken), or if they were added by the copyist. This may have been painted by a Flemish artist in Palermo, possibly Willem Walsgart.

SELECT BIBLIOGRAPHY

Sterling 1939, pp. 59–62; Held 1965, vol. 1, pp. 58–59; Collura 1977, pp. 62, 100; P. Gordon in Princeton 1979, p. 130–31, cat. 35; Larsen 1980a, p. 118, cat. 445; Brown 1982, pp. 81–82; Held 1984, vol. 1, pp. 104–07; Barnes 1986, p. 57 n. 84; Larsen 1988, p. 183, cat. 454; Abbate 1991, p. 95; Bauman and Liedtke 1992, p. 332, cat. 215; Roethlisberger 2002, pp. 98–99; H. Vey in Barnes, De Poorter, Millar, Vey 2004, p. 286, cat. III.51; Bailey 2005, pp. 125–27; M.M. Hale in Phoenix, Memphis and Nashville 2008, pp. 92–93, cat. 28.

EXHIBITIONS

Van Dyck as Religious Artist, The Art Museum, Princeton University, Princeton, New Jersey 1979, cat. 35; *Masterpieces of European Painting from Museo de Arte de Ponce*, Phoenix Art Museum, Phoenix, Memphis Brooks Museum of Art, Memphis and Frist Center for the Visual Arts, Nashville 2008–10, cat. 28.

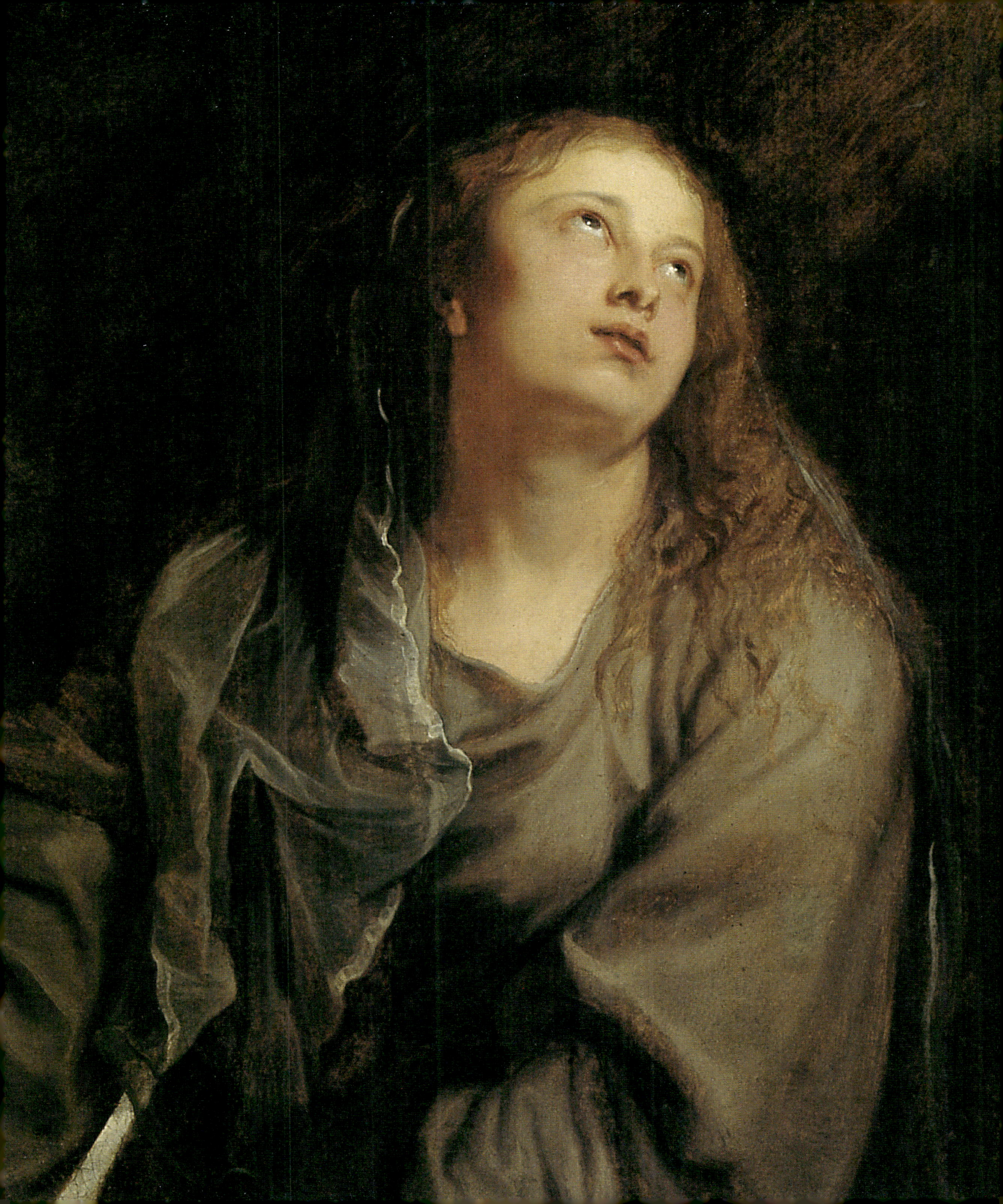

13 | Sir Anthony van Dyck
(1599–1641)

Saint Rosalia Crowned with Roses by Two Angels

c. 1625
Oil on canvas, 117.2 × 88 cm
The Wellington Collection, Apsley House (English Heritage), London
(WM 1651–1948)

PROVENANCE

Palacio Real, Madrid, by 1772; captured by Arthur Wellesley, 1st Duke of Wellington (1769–1852) at the Battle of Vitoria, 1813; donated by King Ferdinand VII of Spain (1784–1833) to the Duke of Wellington, 1816.

The Wellington *Saint Rosalia* is recorded for the first time in the 1772 inventory of the Palacio Real in Madrid, where it was displayed in the 'passage to the king's pew'. Antonio Ponz, in 1776, lists 'two paintings of Saint Rosalia by Van Dyck, very similar one to the other' in the prince's dressing room ('la pieza de vestir el Príncipe') of the Royal Palace. In the inventory of 1789 it was described as a 'Magdalen crowned with roses, in the king's dressing room'. The iconographic confusion continued until 1901, when in the catalogue of the collection of the Duke of Wellington the painting was entitled 'Magdalen with angels (or St. Rosalia?)'.

The canvas was among the two hundred pictures belonging to the Spanish crown that Joseph Bonaparte tried to take with him, and that were found by the Duke of Wellington in Bonaparte's abandoned travelling carriage at the Battle of Vitoria in June 1813. Wellington had the paintings sent to London for safekeeping, and in 1816, the King of Spain, Ferdinand VII, donated them to the duke. Since then the canvas has been displayed at Apsley House, the London residence of the Dukes of Wellington on Hyde Park Corner.

Outside the mouth of the cave on Monte Pellegrino, Rosalia kneels pointing downwards to the landscape, which is probably meant to refer to Palermo. She looks up to heaven, her blonde hair loose over her shoulders, and at her feet are an open book and a skull. The saint wears a brown monastic outfit and holds with her left hand a transparent veil, draped around her shoulders. Two angels enter the painting at top left and one of them holds a lily in his left hand, while with his right he crowns Rosalia with roses.

The painting is a development from La Barbera's image of the saint (cat. 11) and Van Dyck's version of it (cat. 12). It is almost identical in composition to the larger canvas in Houston (cat. 14) of the same subject. The relationship between the London and Houston pictures has been the topic of discussion. According to the majority of art historians, the Wellington *Saint Rosalia* is a first sketchier version, possibly even a finished *modello*, of the Menil painting (Sterling 1939; Kauffmann 1982; Barnes 1986; Bailey 2005; Kauffmann and Jenkins 2009). Julius Held, however, in an unpublished letter to Saemy Rosenberg (of Rosenberg & Stiebel), of 30 March 1963 (conserved in the curatorial files of the Menil Collection in Houston) wrote that 'although Sterling suggests that the version at Apsley House was done before your [Menil] picture, I am inclined to reverse this sequence since the Apsley House picture looks to me somewhat later in style'. There is, however, no reason to doubt that the Wellington canvas preceded the Menil one, and it seems logical that it was a *modello* for it.

Sterling (1939) suggested that this picture may have belonged to Desiderio Segno. It is, however, likely that the canvas belonging to Segno was the one now in The Metropolitan Museum of Art in New York (cat. 16). The London *Saint Rosalia* may be tentatively linked with the one in the 1658 inventory of Marco Gezio (Morreale 1990, p. 44; Mendola 1999b, p. 101; Mendola 1999c, p. 61; Abbate 2004, p. 77); the dimensions given in the document (5 × 4 *palmi* – 129 × 103 cm) are larger, but may have included the frame of the painting. There is not enough evidence to establish what the *Saint Rosalia* recorded in the 1632 inventory of Simone Sitaiolo (Mendola 1999b, p. 101; Mendola 1999c, p. 61; Abbate 2004, p. 74) looked like, or if it could be identified with the Wellington one.

SELECT BIBLIOGRAPHY

Ponz 1776, vol. 6, p. 51; Wellington 1901, vol. 1, pp. 107–08, cat. 246; Glück 1931, p. 156; Sterling 1939, p. 59; Gaya Nuño 1964, p. 44, cat. 138; Collura 1977, pp. 60, 100; P. Gordon in Princeton 1979, pp. 127–28; Larsen 1980a, p. 118, cat. 454; Brown 1982, pp. 81–82; Kauffmann 1982, pp. 53–54, cat. 42; Barnes 1986, p. 57 n. 84, 173–75, cat. 14; Larsen 1988, pp. 182–83, cat. 453; Abbate 1991, p. 95; S.J. Barnes in Barnes, De Poorter, Millar, Vey 2004, p. 160, cat. II.15; Bailey 2005, pp. 127–28; Kauffmann and Jenkins 2009, pp. 102–04, cat. 42.

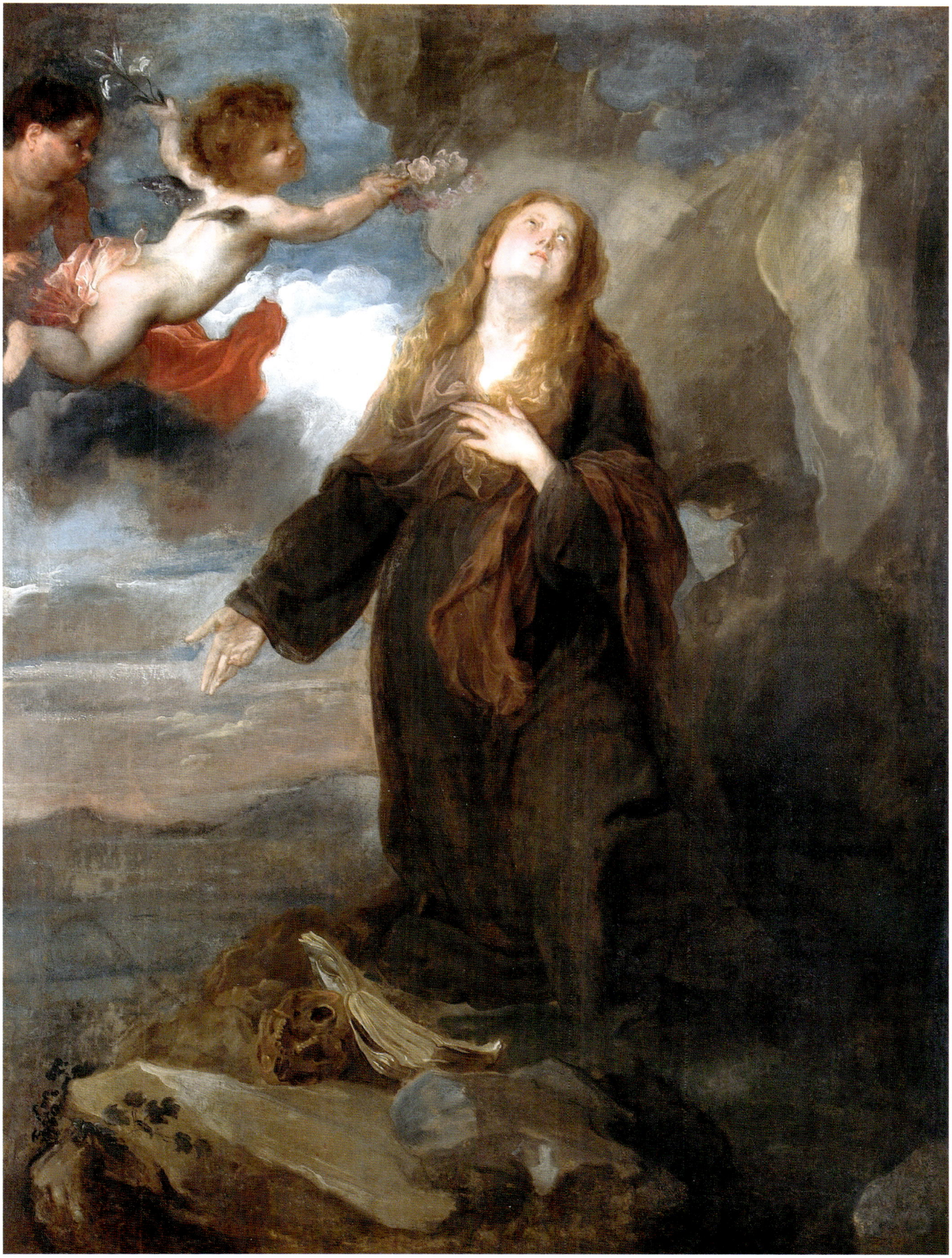

14 | Sir Anthony van Dyck
(1599–1641)

Saint Rosalia Interceding for Palermo

c. 1625
Oil on canvas, 165 × 138 cm
The Menil Collection, Houston
(Inv. 68-01 DJ)

PROVENANCE
Possibly San Pascual Bailon, Madrid, 1776; possibly Manuel de Godoy (1767–1851), Príncipe de la Paz, by 1808; possibly at sale, European Museum, London, (no day given) March 1819 (lot 447); Jean-Gilbert-Victor Fialin, Duc de Persigny (1808–72), by 1866; his sale, Drouot, Paris, 4 April 1872 (lot 7), to M. Gravier; private collection, Paris; sold by Rosenberg & Stiebel, New York, to John (1904–73) and Dominique (1908–97) de Menil, Houston, 1968.

Antonio Ponz, in the fifth volume of his *Viage de España* (1776), describes in the fourth chapel on the right in the church of San Pascual Bailon in Madrid 'an altarpiece with Saint Rosalia, life-size and full-length: which is repeated in a half-length picture in the Chapter House of the Escorial' ('En la quarta Capilla, el quadro del altar es una Santa Rosalía, figura del natural de cuerpo entero: está repetida en un quadro de las salas de Capítuols de Escorial, aunque allí es de medio cuerpo'). The painting at the Escorial is the one from the Museo del Prado in Madrid (cat. 15) and because of its similarity, the picture described by Ponz has been identified with the one in the Menil Collection in Houston, Texas. This may also be the same painting that in 1808 belonged to Manuel de Godoy, Principe de la Paz in Madrid (Rose 1983). The Houston canvas was exhibited with several works from private collections at an exhibition in the Palais des Champs-Elysées in Paris, in May 1866, where it appeared as belonging to the Duc de Persigny, an ardent Bonapartist and supporter of Emperor Napoleon III. Charles Sterling, in 1939, recorded the painting in a Parisian private collection. It was acquired in 1968 by John and Dominique de Menil from the dealers Rosenberg & Stiebel in New York.

The painting is a larger version of the *Saint Rosalia* in the collection of the Duke of Wellington (cat. 13), and the two canvases are almost identical in composition. The figure of the saint was maintained in the same position, outside her cave on Monte Pellegrino; the shape in the Apsley House picture is slightly more elongated. The transparent veil in the London painting was eliminated and substituted with an orange drapery that encircles Rosalia's right arm and wraps around her back, resting on her left knee. She grasps her loose blonde hair at her chest, instead of the veil of the Wellington version. The skull and book were moved to the bottom right corner, and the angel at the top left was changed and now scatters roses onto the landscape below. Julius Held vividly described the painting, in a letter of 30 March 1963 to Saemy Rosenberg (of Rosenberg & Stiebel): 'although a finished painting of impressive size, your canvas preserves in its execution the spirited quality of a sketch [...] the radiantly beautiful Saint in her somberly colored gown holds eloquently the middle between the forces of darkness and of light'.

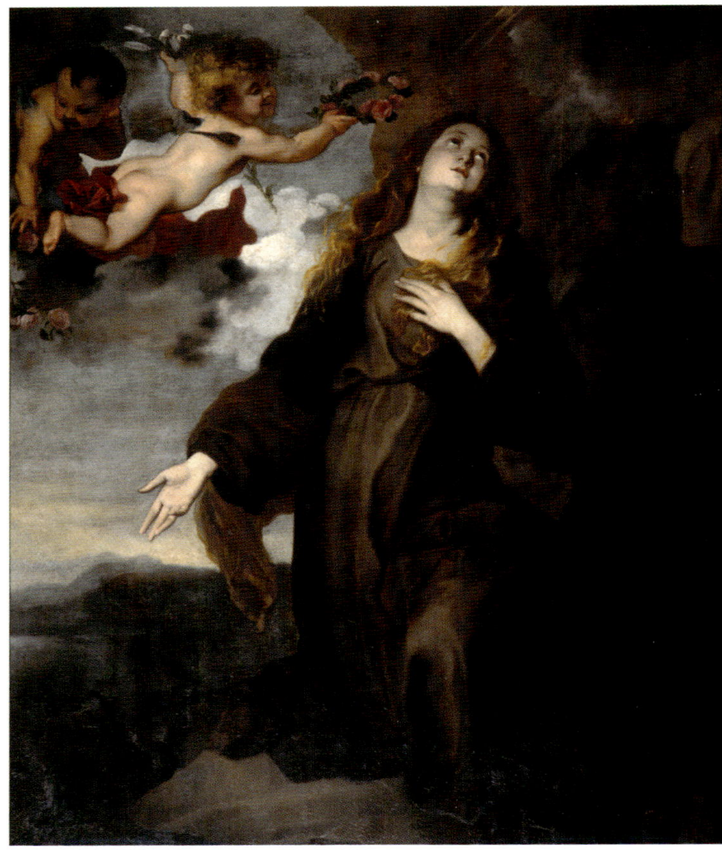

41 | After Sir Anthony van Dyck, *Saint Rosalia Interceding for Palermo*
Galleria Interdisciplinare Regionale della Sicilia di Palazzo Abatellis, Palermo (Inv. 503)

Susan Barnes, in an unpublished letter to Dominique de Menil of 10 August 1984 (the correspondence is in the curatorial file at the Menil Collection, Houston), concluded that the canvas was 'by far the best surviving copy of a lost altarpiece by Van Dyck'; she subsequently published her views in her Ph.D. thesis on Van Dyck's Italian period (1986). Ten years later, however, Barnes revised her opinion. In a letter to Mrs de Menil of 15 June 1995, she wrote 'I now am certain that Charles Sterling was right and I was wrong: it is an autograph work by Van Dyck'. Barnes explained her doubts in the painting, caused by certain unusual compositional features: 'in my opinion she was painted to be placed over an altar on the right wall of a chapel. This explains the "awkwardnesses" I noted in the artist's rendering of the proper left side of her body and the skull in the foreground; they are foreshortened for an angular point of view, from the altar rail that would have enclosed the chapel space. The large scale and placement of the left leg also make it serve as a repoussoir and enhance the feeling that Rosalie is tall and drawn heavenward.'

There is no evidence of the original patron of the canvas, as its first documented reference is in 1866. While Barnes's suggestion that the painting was made as an altarpiece for the right wall of a chapel is plausible, there is no substantiation that Van Dyck was commissioned a public work of this kind. The canvas is more likely to have been a devotional painting intended for a pri-

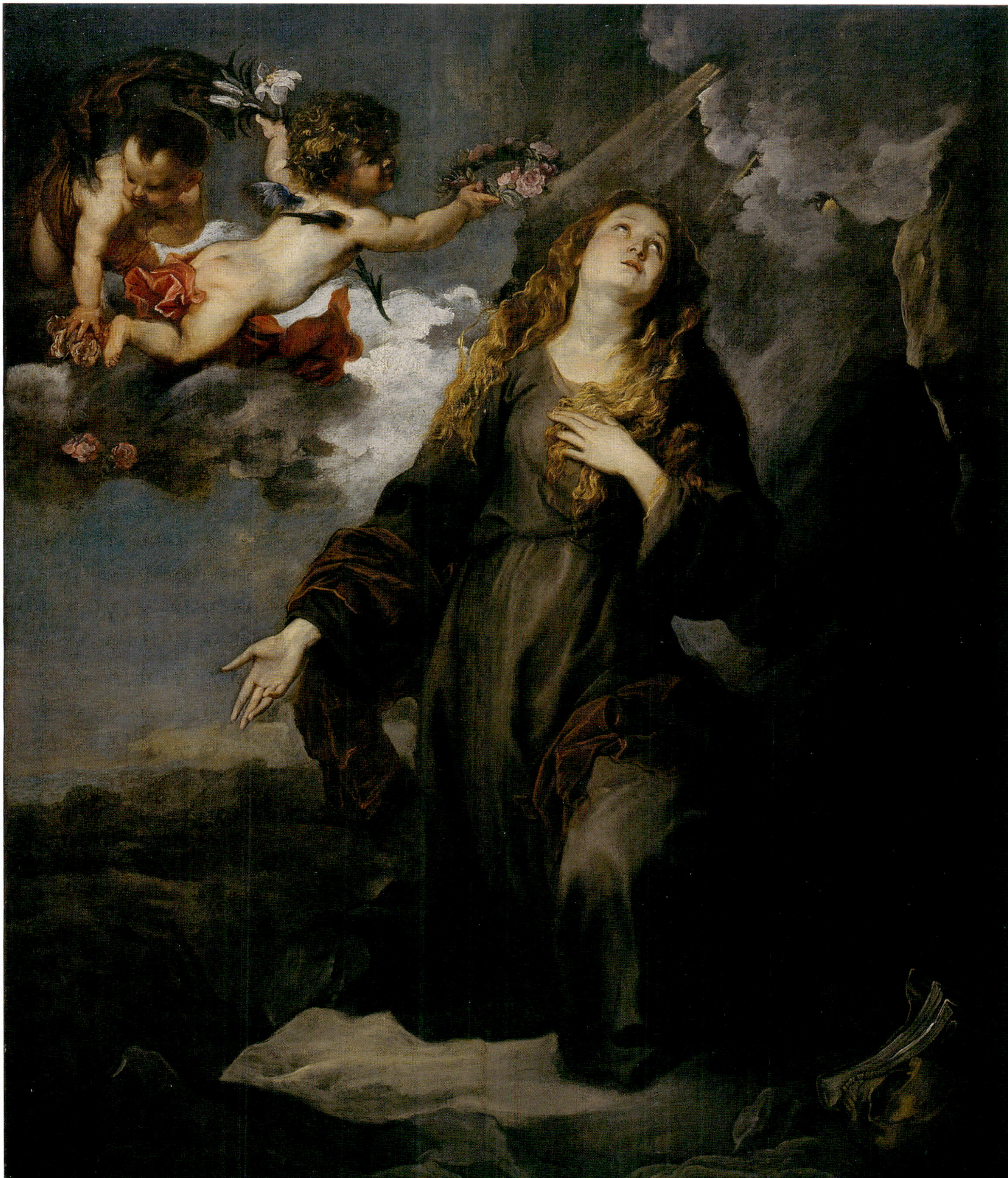

vate individual. Sterling (1939), hypothesised that either the Houston or the London *Saint Rosalia* was painted for Desiderio Segno, but it is now believed that Segno's canvas is the one in New York (cat. 16); Gordon (1979) also tentatively connected the Menil picture with Segno's.

Van Dyck's half-length of *Saint Rosalia* in the Prado (cat. 15) is particularly close in composition and style to the London and Houston paintings. A half-length copy of the Menil picture was formerly in the collection of Harry Axelson Johnson in Stockholm. Another, full-length, slightly smaller (156 × 126 cm) copy from the Belmonte collection, is now in the Galleria Regionale in Palermo, and may be the work of Willem Walsgart (fig. 41 – Matranga 1908, pp. 13–14; D. Bernini in Palermo 1990a, pp. 176–80, cat. 31).

SELECT BIBLIOGRAPHY

Ponz 1776, vol. 5, p. 39; Guiffrey 1882, p. 252, cat. 213; Sterling 1939, p. 59; Houston 1968, cat. 67; Collura 1977, p. 100; P. Gordon in Princeton 1979, pp. 127–29, cat. 34; Larsen 1980a, p. 118, cat. 443; Brown 1982, pp. 81–82; Rose 1983, vol. 2, pp. 118–20; Barnes 1986, pp. 57 n. 84, 347–49, cat. B2; Larsen 1988, pp. 181–82, cat. 451; Abbate 1991, p. 95; S.J. Barnes in Barnes, De Poorter, Millar, Vey 2004, p. 161, cat. II.16; Bailey 2005, p. 127; G.A. Bailey in Worcester 2005, pp. 236–37, cat. 30.

EXHIBITIONS

Retrospective Exhibition, Palais des Champs-Elysées, Paris 1866, cat. 45; *A Young Teaching Collection*, Museum of Fine Arts, Houston 1968–69, cat. 67; *Devotional Art of Living Religions*, Museum of Fine Arts, Houston 1971, cat. 8; *Selections from the Menil Collection*, Institute for the Arts, Rice University, Houston 1971–72; *Antwerp's Golden Age*, Institute for the Arts, Rice University, Houston 1975; *Rubens and his Circle*, Art History Galleries, University of Wisconsin, Milwaukee 1977; *Art Survey: The Real Thing*, Institute for the Arts, Rice University, Houston 1978; *Van Dyck as Religious Artist*, The Art Museum, Princeton University, Princeton, New Jersey 1979, cat. 34; *Time after Time*, Sewall Art Gallery, Rice University, Houston 1981; *Hope and Healing: Paintings in Italy in a Time of Plague, 1500–1800*, Worcester Art Museum, Worcester Massachusetts 2005, cat. 30.

Saint Rosalia Interceding for Palermo, detail (cat. 14)

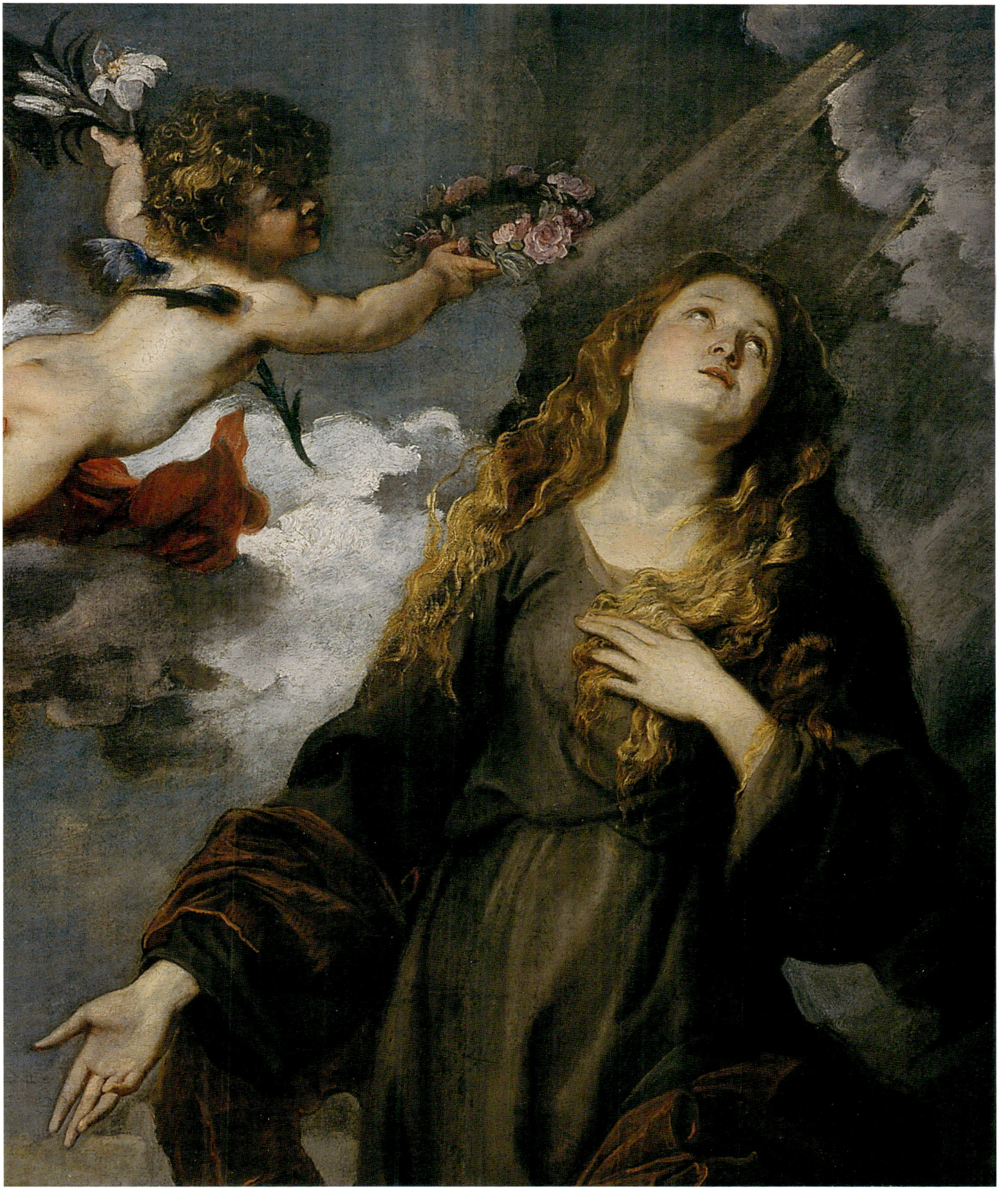

15 | Sir Anthony van Dyck
(1599–1641)

Saint Rosalia

c. 1625
Oil on canvas, 106 × 81 cm
Museo Nacional del Prado, Madrid
(Inv. PO 1494)

PROVENANCE

Giovan Francesco Serra di Cassano (1609–56), Genoa and Naples; sold to King Philip IV of Spain (1605–65) through Gaspar de Bracamonte y Guzmán, Conde de Peñaranda (1596–1676), Viceroy of Naples, 1664; Spanish Royal Collection, El Escorial, since at least 1667; Museo del Prado, Madrid, from 1839.

This painting of *Saint Rosalia* is recorded in 1664 in the inventory of the paintings that had belonged to the Marchese Giovan Francesco Serra di Cassano in Genoa and that his heirs were selling in Naples to King Philip IV of Spain, through the mediation of the Viceroy of Naples, the Conde de Peñaranda. It is described as 'a Saint Rosalia half figure by Anthony van Dyck, 4 ¼ *palmi* high and 3 ½ wide' ('1 S.ta Rosolea mezza figura d'Ant.o vandich alto p.mi 4 ¼, e 3 ½' – Vannugli 1989, p. 74). As soon as the painting entered the Spanish Royal Collection it was displayed at El Escorial, where Francisco de los Santos (1667) records it two years later. The canvas was displayed in one of the Chapter Rooms, in the 'Capitulo del Vicario', over a door, as a pendant to the *Ecce Homo with Saint Peter* attributed to Titian, and two still lifes with flowers ('floreros') by Daniel Seghers. The painting of the same subject, listed in the 1686 inventory of the Alcázar in Madrid ('Otra Pintura en Lienço sin marco de Santa Rosolea de vara y quarta de alto por adreçar de mano de Bandique') as one of the 'pinturas desmontadas' in the 'cuarto bajo del Príncipe' (Bottineau 1958, p. 478, cat. 1507) has been identified as the work in the Escorial. It has been suggested that this was moved temporarily to Madrid for restoration but, as proved by Vannugli, these are two different paintings. The Escorial canvas was transferred to the Prado in 1839.

The smallest of the paintings of Saint Rosalia produced by Van Dyck in Sicily, this is a devotional image for an unknown patron. The composition is similar to the canvases in London (cat. 13) and Houston (cat. 14), with the face of Rosalia looking up to heaven. She is portrayed in her cave on Monte Pellegrino, while an angel offers her a crown of roses. Her right hand is to her breast, while the left holds a skull. A copy of the painting is in the Galleria Regionale della Sicilia in Palermo (Collura 1977, p. 100).

SELECT BIBLIOGRAPHY

De los Santos 1667, p. 77; Ximenez 1764, p. 97; Bermejo 1820, p. 202 n. 21; Sánchez Cantón 1933, vol. 2, pp. 303–04; *Catalogo* 1952, p. 185, cat. 1494; Du Gué Trapier 1957, p. 273; Bottineau 1958, p. 478, cat. 1507; De Andrés 1971, p. 54; Collura 1977, p. 100; Larsen 1980a, p. 188, cat. 452; Barnes 1986, p. 380; Larsen 1988, p. 184, cat. 455; Vannugli 1989, pp. 15, 37–39, 74–76; Abbate 1991, p. 95; Bailey 2005, p. 130.

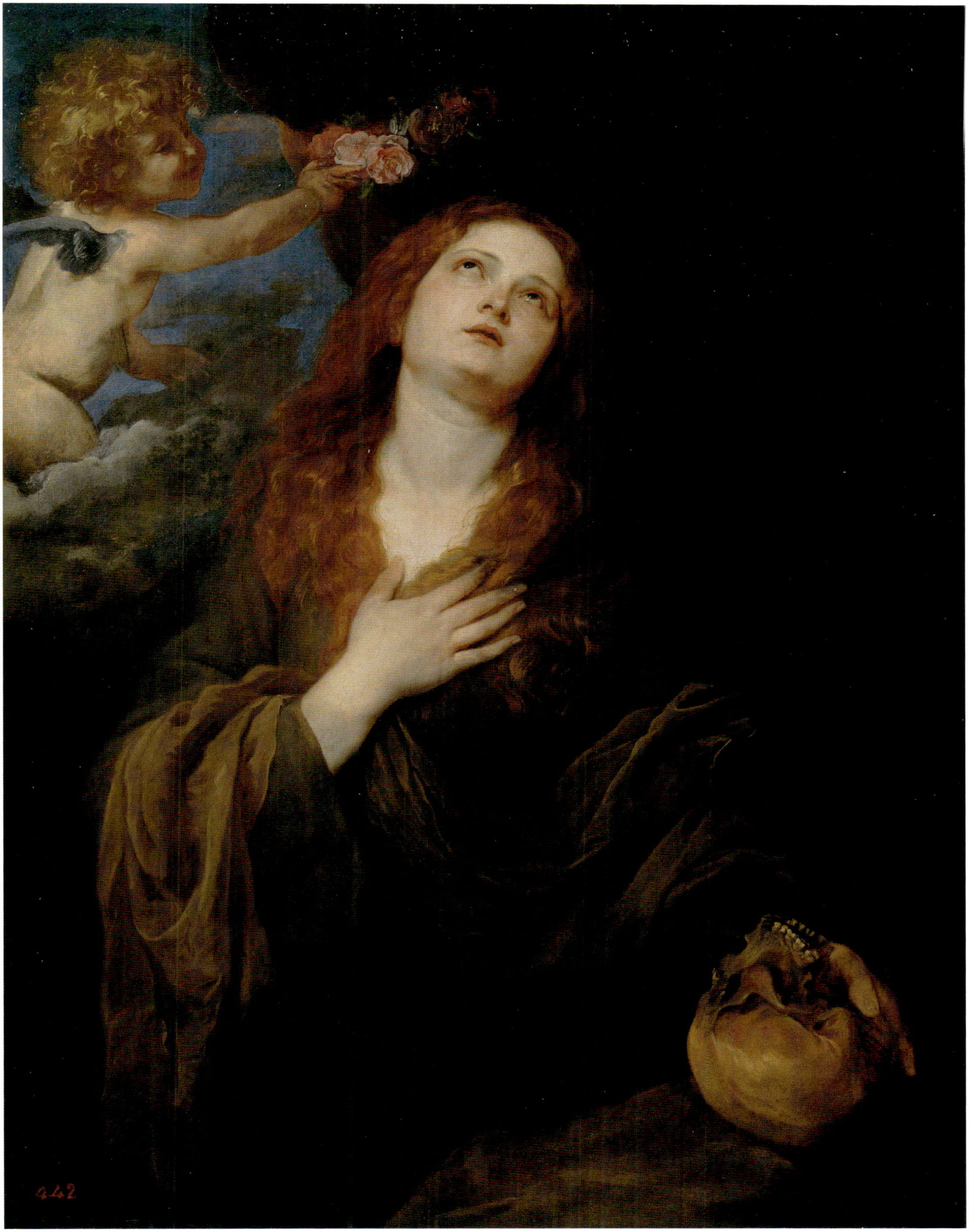
442

16 | Sir Anthony van Dyck
(1599–1641)

Saint Rosalia in Glory Interceding for Palermo

c. 1625
Oil on canvas, 99.7 × 73.7 cm
The Metropolitan Museum of Art, New York
Purchase, 1871 (71.41)

PROVENANCE

Possibly Desiderio Segno (d. 1630), Palermo and Salaparuta, 1630; don Antonio Ruffo (1610/11–1678), Principe della Scaletta, Messina, bought by 25 April 1648; by descent in the Ruffo family until after 1750; Thomas Emmerson, London; his sale, Phillips, London, 1 May 1829 (lot 84); possibly D.M. Farrer, London; David McIntosh (d. 1857), London; his sale, Christie's, London, 16 May 1857 (lot 65); C.J. Nieuwenhuys, London and Brussels; Marquise Théodule de Rodes (d. 1867); her sale, Hôtel Drouot, Paris, 30 May 1868 (lot 4); Prince Paskiewitz; Étienne Le Roy, Brussels, through Léon Gauchez, Paris; William T. Blodgett (1823–75), Paris and New York; half-share bought by John Taylor Johnston (1820–93), 1870; William T. Blodgett and John Taylor Johnston, New York, 1871; sold to the Metropolitan Museum of Art, New York 1871.

Don Antonio Ruffo, one of the most important Sicilian collectors of the seventeenth century, acquired Van Dyck's *Saint Rosalia* in Palermo in 1648. It is recorded in his expense book of 1644–55 where it is described as 'a painting by Anthony van Dyck, Flemish, of 3 by 4 ½ *palmi*, bought in Palermo, with a Saint Rosalia and eleven small angels, that carry her into heaven, it cost 26 *onze*, and 3 *onze* for the frame, and 1 *onza* for the crate and its rental, for a total of 30 *onze*' ('È p. uno quadro di Ant.o Vandijck fiam.go di p.mi 3 e 4 ½ Comp.to In Pal.mo Con una S.ta Rosolea e undici Angioletti che la tirano In Cielo, costò oz. 26 – e oz. 3 p. la cornizza È oz. una p. la Cassa e Nolo In tutto oz. 30 dico quadro n.ro 1 Oz. 30', Ruffo 1916, p. 29). The receipt for the painting was signed on 25 April 1648: '*onze* 26 are for the price of a painting sent to me, by the hand of Van Dyck, bought through the above said Prossimi, with a Saint Rosalia and twelve angels, as in his letter of 10 of this April' ('A 25 detto [aprile 1648] E onze 26 – sono per Prezzo d'un quadro mandatomi di Mano del Vandich fiamingo comprato per mano del predetto Prussimi con una Santa Rosolia e dodeci Puttini come con sua lettera delli 10 dell'Istante ap.re', Ruffo 1919, p. 46). The canvas was acquired through the mediation of one of Ruffo's agents, don Antonino Prossimi, originally from Messina, who served Ruffo's interests in Palermo.

The painting subsequently appears in the Ruffo inventories of 1 January 1652, 1 January 1668, and in an undated one in 1677 (De Gennaro 2003), and later in more inventories of 6 July 1678, 23 January 1703 and 31 December 1739 (Ruffo 1916, p. 33 n. 1). In 1908, discussing the Metropolitan's *Saint Rosalia*, Sidney J.A. Churchill first mentioned the painting of the same subject that appeared in the *post-mortem* inventory, of 24 December 1630, of Desiderio Segno's collection, but did not connect the two directly. Vincenzo Abbate (1999b, p. 113) has reasonably proposed that Segno's *Saint Rosalia*, described as 'a painting of Saint Rosalia in glory, by Anthony van Dyck, with a black frame' ('un quatro di S. Rosalia in gloria, di mano di Antonio Vandich, con guarnizione negra', Di Giovanni 1889, p. 288), is the same canvas that Ruffo bought in Palermo in 1648. Out of all the surviving images of Rosalia by Van Dyck, this is the only one that could truly be described as 'in gloria'. The painting remained in the Ruffo family until after 1750 and next appeared at the sale of Thomas Emmerson's collection in London in May 1829. After having passed through various aristocratic collections in London, Brussels and Paris, the canvas was bought for The Metropolitan Museum of Art in 1871.

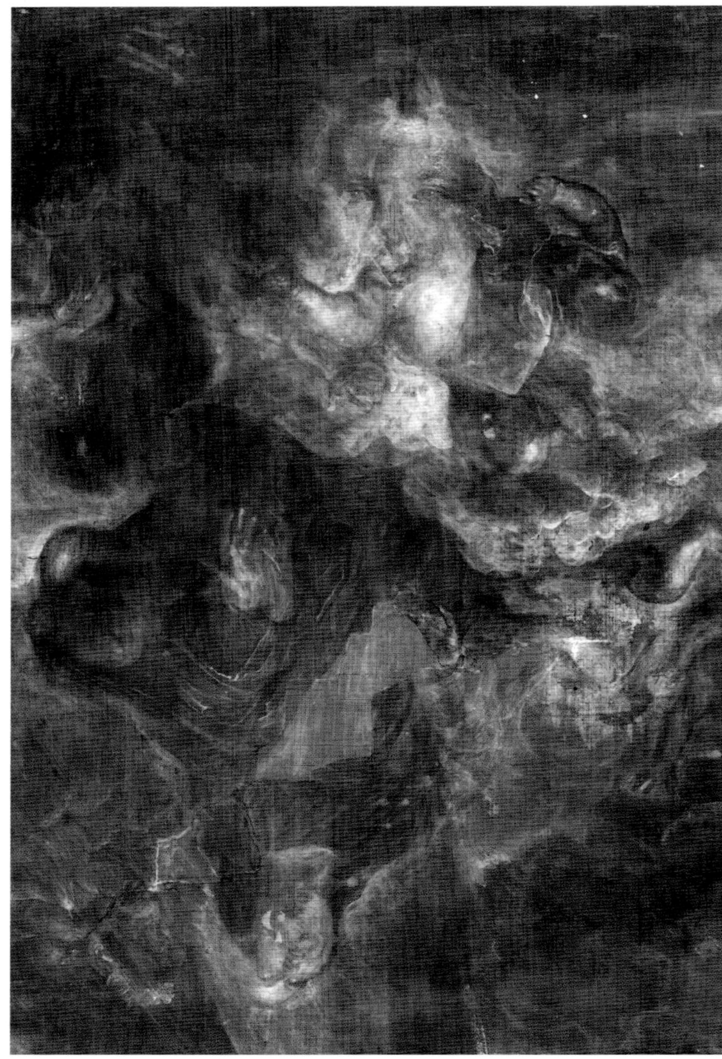

42 | Sir Anthony van Dyck, X-ray of *Saint Rosalia in Glory Interceding for Palermo*
The Metropolitan Museum of Art, New York

The subject of the painting was misinterpreted for a long time. In the London auction catalogues of Emmerson's (1829) and of David McIntosh's collections (1857) the picture was described as 'The Assumption of the Virgin'. It was also mistakenly given a provenance 'from the King of Spain's Collection' (1829) or 'from the Royal Gallery of Madrid' (1857). This erroneous provenance (repeated, for example, in Gaya Nuño 1964, p. 44, cat. 139, and in Larsen 1988, p. 181) was caused by the presence of a larger copy of the New York painting in the Spanish Royal Collection and now in the Museo del Prado (127 × 108 cm – see Larsen

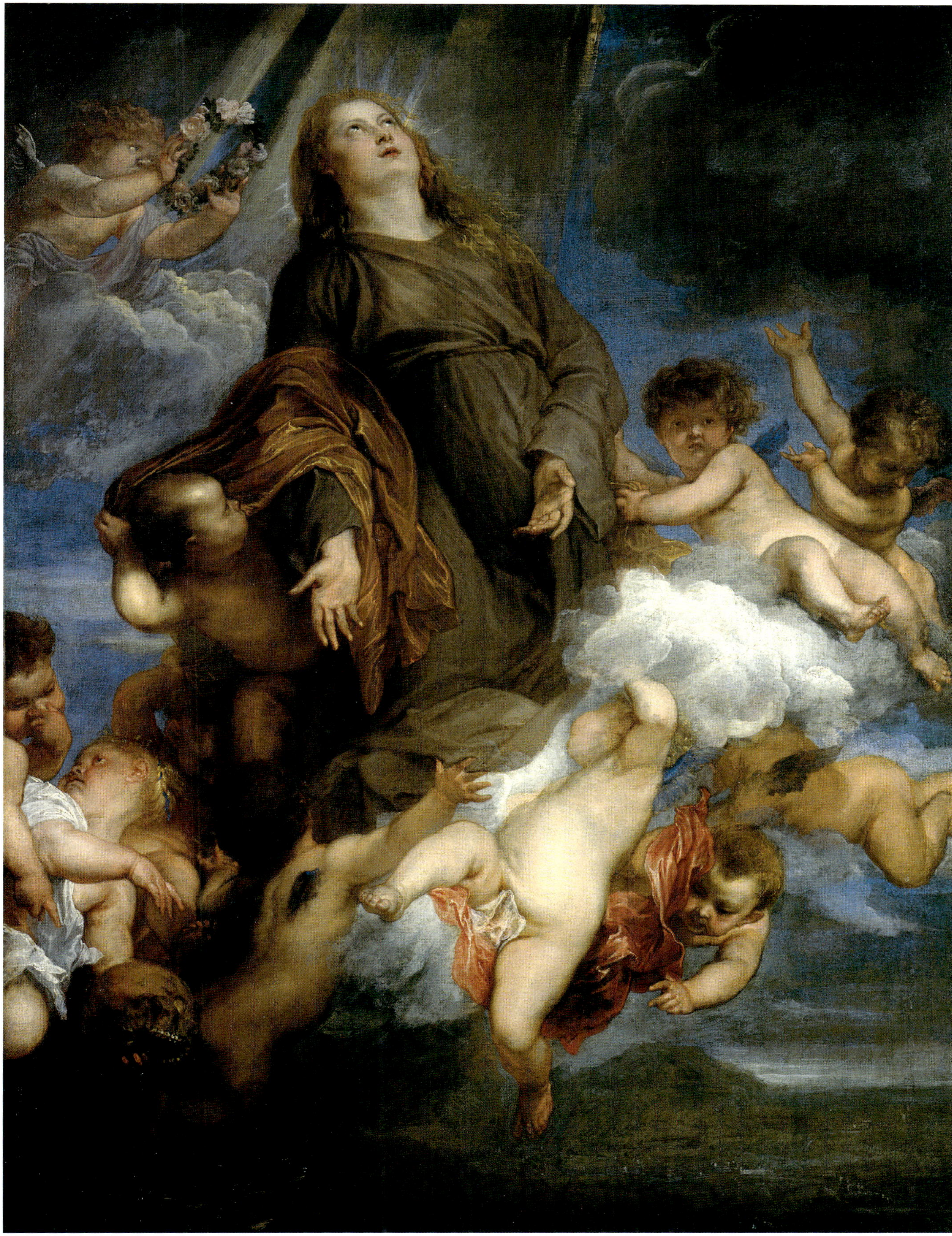

1980a, p. 118, cat. 451). By the time the canvas was listed in the auction catalogue of the pictures of the Marquise Théodule de Rodes, in Paris in 1868, it was described as 'Sainte Marthe Implorant le Christ en Faveur des Habitants de Tarascon', and this was repeated in the Metropolitan's catalogue of 1872: 'Saint Martha interceding with God for a cessation of the Plague in Tarascon'. Henry James, in the same year, wrote about the 'Saint Martha' and 'the lovely flesh-glow of the tumbling cherubs who uplift the pretty postulant into the blue, and who form, with the warm purple of her robe, the main success of the picture' (James 1956, p. 55). It was Gustav Glück, in 1931, who first identified the saint as Rosalia and connected the painting in New York with the reference in Ruffo's documents.

X-radiography shows that Van Dyck painted *Saint Rosalia* over an already used canvas, where he had painted a *Self-Portrait*, probably the only one made while he was in Sicily (fig. 42). The composition of the painting is particularly close to images of the *Assumption of the Virgin* – hence the wrong description in the 1829 and 1857 auction catalogues – and in particular to Van Dyck's later *Assumption*, of around 1630, in the National Gallery of Art, Washington (H. Vey in Barnes, De Poorter, Millar, Vey 2004, pp. 274–75, cat. III.37). Rosalia is depicted in the same outfit as in the Houston painting (cat. 14), with the brown dress and orange shawl. She gazes up as she is carried into heaven by a group of angels on clouds. At the top left an angel offers her a crown of roses; another angel below holds a skull. The angel next to the latter points downward and holds his nose, in a manner often connected to plague-related images, and which Van Dyck also used in his *Madonna of the Rosary* (fig. 33). Below the group is a view of the city of Palermo with Monte Pellegrino in the background.

Copies of the painting were in the Spanish Royal Collection (now at the Museo Nacional del Prado, Madrid) and in the Electoral Gallery in Düsseldorf (now at the Alte Pinakothek in Munich). A copy on copper is in the Galleria Regionale di Sicilia in Palermo.

SELECT BIBLIOGRAPHY

Catalogue 1872, p. 12, cat. 5; Churchill 1908, pp. 239–40; Ruffo 1916, pp. 29, 33, 42, 320; Ruffo 1919, pp. 46–47; Glück 1931, pp. 536–37; Sterling 1939, p. 54; Genoa 1955, pp. 31–32, cat. 54; James 1956, p. 55; Montebello 1963, p. 138; Gaya Nuño 1964, p. 44, cat. 139; Collura 1977, p. 100; P. Gordon in Princeton 1979, p. 125; Larsen 1980a, pp. 117–18, cat. 442; Ainsworth 1982, pp. 12–18, 101–03; Brown 1982, pp. 81–82; Liedtke 1984a, pp. 43–48; Liedtke 1984b, pp. 26–30; Barnes 1986, pp. 56, 170–71, cat. 13; Larsen 1988, p. 181, cat. 449; Abbate 1991, p. 95; Moir 1994, p. 80; Abbate 1999b, p. 113; Giltaij 1999, pp. 19, 25, 102–03; De Gennaro 2003, pp. 69–70, 107, 126, nos. 322, 483, 587; Baetjer 2004, pp. 164, 169–70, 172, 178, 183, 192–93, 197–98, 244–45; S.J. Barnes in Barnes, De Poorter, Millar, Vey 2004, pp. 159–60, cat. II.14; M.G. Bernardini in Milan 2004, p. 162, cat. 11; Bailey 2005, pp. 128–29; G.A. Bailey in Worcester 2005, pp. 238–39, cat. 31; W. Prohaska in Naples 2007, pp. 156–57, cat. 68; Abbate 2011, pp. 95–96.

EXHIBITIONS

The Taste of the Seventies, The Metropolitan Museum of Art, New York 1946, cat. 10; *100 Opere di Van Dyck*, Palazzo dell'Accademia, Genoa 1955, cat. 54; *Exhibition from The Metropolitan Museum of Art*, Union League Club, New York 1969–70, cat. 11; *Spectrum: A Cross Section from the Metropolitan Museum of Art, New York*, Fort Worth Art Center Museum, Fort Worth, Texas 1970; *Anthony van Dyck*, Sogo Museum of Art, Yokohama, Shizuoka Prefectural Museum of Art, Shizuoka, and Museum of Art, Kintetsu, Osaka 1990, cat. 9; *From El Greco to Cézanne: Masterpieces of European Painting from the National Gallery of Art, Washington, and The Metropolitan Museum of Art, New York*, National Gallery Alexandros Soutzos Museum, Athens 1992–93, cat. 9; *Anton van Dyck: Riflessi italiani*, Palazzo Reale, Milan 2004, cat. 11; *Hope and Healing. Painting in Italy in a Time of Plague 1500–1800*, Worcester Art Museum, Worcester, Massachusetts 2005, cat. 31; *Omaggio a Capodimonte: da Caravaggio a Picasso*, Museo di Capodimonte, Naples 2007–08, cat. 68.

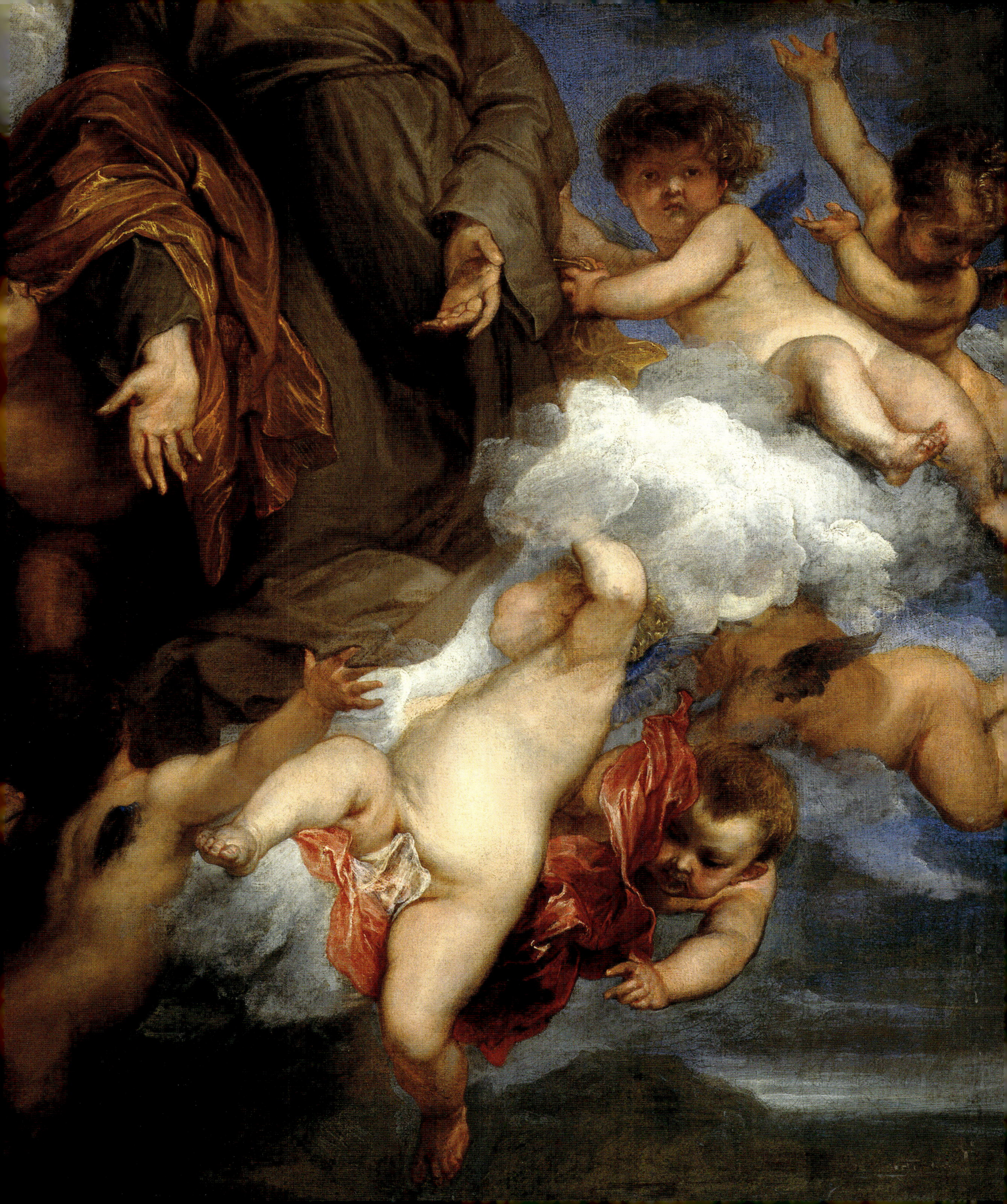

Appendices and bibliography

Appendix 1

Regulations against the spread of the plague (1624–26) from *Raccolta di originali scritture e stampe sulla peste di Palermo degli anni 1624 e 1625, oltre alcune di altre pestilenze*, Biblioteca Comunale, Palermo, Ms. Qq H 59

Doc. 1

Editto. Poi che il Sig. Iddio s'è compiaciuto ad intercessione della sua gloriosissima Vergine SANTA ROSALIA Patrona e Cittadina di Palermo, di liberar' affatto questa Città dal morbo contagioso, per il che si spera con la divina gratia il dì della viglia della sua festa dar la prattica e libero commercio per tutti; volendo l'Illustrissimo e Reverendissimo Signor Cardinal' Arcivescovo che in memoria di tal beneficio, se ne faccia alcuna dimostrazione, per il presente Editto ordina, provede, e comanda che il giorno della festa di detta Santa, che farà alli 4. di Settembre sia perpetuamente guardato da tutti Fedeli tanto nella Città, quant'ancora nel Territorio di essa, come qualsivoglia altra festa di precetto, obligando tutti, e qualsivoglia persona à udir Messa, & astenersi dalle opere servili. Et affinche nel present'anno, nel quale habbiam ricevuto la liberatione dal contagio, si rendano al Signore le dovute gratie; Ordina S.S. Illustrissima, che per questa volta tantum il Mercordi prossimo che saranno li 3. del presente Mese, s'habbia a far la vigilia di detta festa con digiuno ecclesiastico, come nell'altre vigilie di precetto, esortando tutti che in segno di riconoscimento ricevano il Santis. Sacramento dell'Eucaristia doppo d'haver fatto un'esatta confessione de' loro peccati. E per venir à notitia di tutti s'è fatto quest'Editto, e s'è attaccato alli luoghi pubblici, e consueti della Città. Dat. in Pal. Nel Palazzo Arcives. il 1. di Settembre 1625

Doc. 2

Editto. Considerando l'Illustrissimo e Reverendissimo Signor Cardinal Doria Arcivescovo di Palermo che quantunque si debba sperare la liberatione del morbo contagioso per l'intercessione della gloriosa SANTA ROSALIA Patrona, e Cittadina di questa Città; non per questo si debbono lasciar da parte li mezzi e diligenze humane, per non dilatarsi il male con l'occasione d'aggiuntarsi insieme tanta gente, ha deliberato a commun' sodisfattione, e consolatione del Populo Palermitano, di lasciar' il suo Santo Corpo esposto nella Chiesa Cattedrale per 8. giorni continui, fatta che sarà la procession' sollenne, nelle quali potrà andare tutta la gente di Palermo ad adorarlo, diviso per giornate nelli quattro quarti della Città. Dio maniera che quelli che habitano nel quarto chiamato di S. Cristina, Huomini come Donne anderanno il Martedi seguente, & il Sabbato che saranno li 10. e 14. del presente mese di Giugno: quelli del quarto di S. Nimfa, il Mercordi, e la Domenica, cioè adi 11. & adi 15. quelli del quarto di S. Agata Giovedi, e lunidi, cioè adi 12. & adi 16. e quelli del quarto di S. Oliva Venerdi e Martedi, cioè adi 13. e 17. Di detto mese; dispensando Sua Signoria Illustrissima per quest'effetto a tutti gl'ordini in contrario, & editti per li quali si comanda che le Donne vadano alla Chiesa più vicina. E perciò s'ordina che fuori delle sudette giornate secondo la presente divisione nissuna persona di qualsivoglia stato, sesso, e condition' si sia la qual' habita in uno delli detti quarti della Città, possa sotto qualunque prestesto entrare nella Chiesa Cattedrale in giorno ch'entrano quelli d'un altro quarto senza particolar' licenza di Sua Signoria Illustrissima sotto pena di Scomunica maggiore latae sententiae ipso facto incurrenda, & altre pene ardue a Sua Signoria Illustrissima benviste, le quali infallibilmente s'eseguiranno. Per il che s'è pubblicato il presente editto, per venir' a notitia di tutti, e per esortarli ancora che in 'tutto questo tempo ciascuno deve procurare portars'in maniera, che muova il Signor Iddio per mezzo di Santissimi Sacramenti, e vera penitenza, ad haver pieta del suo afflitto populo, e che a intercessione di questa Gloriosissima Santa Cittadina e Patrona di Palermo, le conceda hormai la desiderata salute dell'anime e de' corpi. Dat. in Palermo nel Palazzo Arcivescovale adi 6. di Giugno 1625

Doc. 3

D. Gioannettino Doria Prete Cardinale della Santa Romana Chiesa del Tit. di San Pietro Montorio, & Arcivescovo di Palermo, al suo dileto Populo salute.

Havendo ultimamente pubblicato un Editto a 17 del mese di Dicembre pross. pals. Nel quale si comandò che tutte le persone di qualsivoglia stato, grado, sesso, e conditione, rivelassero la robba infetta o sospetta, o le persone che la tenessero a Noi, o nostro Vicario Generale, fra termino di giorni 8. altrimenti haveressimo proceduto contra di loro, con fulminar sentenza di scommunica maggiore, dichiarandoli nella Cattedrale, nelle Parrocchiali, e nell'altre chiese della Città per iscommunicati, e membri putridi di Santa Chiesa, come nel sudetto Editto si contiene; Adesso dichiariamo che già il detto termine di giorni 8. assegnato per trina, e canonica monitione è perento, & elasso, e che è spirata ancora la prorogatione che s'è concessa' e perciò tutte quelle persone che sono state disobedienti, e contumaci sono già incorse nella detta scommunica; la qual dichiaratione e publicatione, habbiam' ordinato che si faccia solennemente; Cioè con spargersi l'acqua benedetta † in segno di cacciar' i demonij, che tengono legate queste tali persone con suoi lacci, e catene: con leggersi il Salmo Deus laudem meam ne tacueris, con l'antifona Media vita &c. e col responsor. Revelabunt &c. in legno che sono maledetti, & incorsi nell'ira di Dio onnipotente, della sua Santissima Madre sempre Vergine Maria, delli Santi Apostoli Pietro, e Paolo, e di tutti Santi, e Sante della Corte celestiale (a) con smorzarsi le candele nell'acqua, in segno che come muoiono le candele nell'acqua, cosi saran sepolte le lor'Anime nell'Inferno (b) e con suonar le campane, ch'è la cerimonia solita usarsi, in queste occasioni di scommuniche; (c) Annuntiandoli che verranno sopra di esse, & ogn'una di loro tutte le maledittioni, e piaghe d'Egitto, che vennero sopra il Re Pharaone e la sua gente, per non haver' obedito alli comandamenti di Dio, e se l'aggiongerà la sentenza di Sodoma, Gomorra, Dathan, & Abiron, li quali furono brugiati vivi per l'inobedienza che commesero contra Dio Nostro Signore: saranno queste persone, & ogn'una di loro maledette nel mangiar' e bevere, nel vegliare, e dormire, nel levarsi di letto, e camminare, nel campar' e morire: il Diavolo starrà appresso di loro, e nel tempo del giuditio, saran condennate: i lor giorni saran pochi, e mali: la robba e li beni saran trasferiti a stranieri; i figli saran orfani e bisognosi; le case, & habitationi brugiate: saran aborriti di maniera che non troveran persona, ch'abbia compassione di lor' o di lor figli: la malignità loro starà continuamente nel cospetto di Dio: le sarà maladetto il pane e'l vino, la carne, i pesci, e tutto quanto mangiaranno e beveranno: le vesti che vestiranno, & il letto dove dormiranno, saran maledetti, con tutte le maledittioni, del vecchio, e nuovo testamento; saran maledetti con Lucifero, e Giuda e con tutti li Diavoli dell'Inferno, li quali staranno in lor compagnia. Laonde comandamo a tutti Confessori secolari, e regolari, che non diano, a queste tali persone il benefitio dell'assoluzione, la quale riserbiamo a Noi stessi, & esortiamo tutti fedeli Cristiani, che voglin pregare Nostro Signore Giesù Christo sia servito ridurle all'unione della Santa Madre Chiesa Romana, e non permetta per sua infinita misericordia che muoiano in tal'ostinatione, e perversità. Amen. In Palermo, Adi 4. di Gennaro 1626.

Appendix 2

Inventory of Desiderio Segno, 24 December 1630. *Inventario degli oggetti mobili rinvenuti nella casa mortuaria di d. Desiderio Segnio, estratto dall'atto compilato dal Notaro Pietro Lombardo di Salaparuta, nel dì 24 dicembre 1630* *

1 In primis una catina di oro smaltata fatta atocca di pezzi N. 150, di peso 11 unzi, et mezza, et menza quarta
2 Un'altra catina di oro smaltata piccola di pezzi 107, di peso di tri unzi, et menza quarta
3 Un'altra catina di oro liscia, di magli 313, di peso di ottu unzi et menza, et menza quarta
4 Una golera di oro con diamanti ingastati di N. 32 et di peso di unza una et menza, et menza quarta
5 Un anello di oro, con uno diamante ingastato, rotto in due pezzi, di peso di menza quarta, et diciottu cocci
6 Un paro di manigli di oro, con diamanti ingastati, di N. 16 quali sono di peso di dui unzi e tri quarti, et vinti cocci
7 Un paru di pindagli di oro con diamandi di N. 14, et di piso di tre quarti et vinti cocci
8 Un anello di oro con un diamanti, di peso di menza quarta, et trenta cocci
10 Un agnusedeo do oro con figuri, di peso di un'unza, et tri quarti, et menza; compresi li cristalli et figuri
11 Una rusetta di oro, con diamanti di N. 17; et di peso di menza unza
12 Una rusetta di diamanti piccoli di N. 9, fatta in anello, di peso di menza quarta
13 Una buttunera di oro smaltati, di butuni N. 43, di peso di unza una, et menza, et tri quarti
14 Uno cintiglio di oro di coppella, di pezzi ottanta, piccoli, smaltati, di peso di unza una, et menza quarta con tutta la cinturetta
15 Buttuna di oro N. 49 smaltati et intagliati, di peso di once cinque
16 Un anello di oro con uno rubino ingastato di peso di menza quarta, et vinti cocci
17 Un altro anello di oro con un topazio ingastato, di peso di menza quarta
18 Un paro di pendagli di oro, con rubini ingastati di N. 6 con 14 perli, di peso onza 1
19 Un altro paro di pendagli di corallo con oro, di peso una quarta, et menza, et 20 cocci
20 Un anello di oro con tri adamantine, di peso di 40 cocci
21 Due rusetti piccoli di ori per orecchini senza pendagli, con diamanti di N. 18 et di peso di menza unza, manco 20 cocci
22 Una crucetta di oro, con ametisti, di peso tri quarti
23 Un anello di oro con uno ismiraldo, et con 12 diamantini ingastati a torno, di peso di una quarta et menza, e 30 cocci
24 Un anello di oro, fatto a [...] smaltato di negro, con 7 diamantini ingastati di peso di menza quarta
25 Un agnus dei di oro piccolo, di peso di unza una, compresi li caristalli e li figuri
26 Un anilluzzo di oro per figliolo, con diamantine di N. 8 et di peso menza quarta
27 Un paio di manigli di oro piccoli smaltati, di peso di unza una, et tri quarti
28 Una collana di coralli di pezzi 98, di peso di 11 unzi, et menza
29 Un paio di pindagli di pasta di oduri, legati con oro, di peso di una quarta
30 Uno paviglıuni grandi di damasco chermisino, in tri pezzi, con suo cappello, tornialetto, et cultra, et dui portali dello stesso damasco, colli suoi finzi di oro
31 Uno paviglıuni virdi et giarno, di sita, et capicciola
32 Uno paviglioni di taffità giarno, con sua cultra, et tornialetto
33 Uno cortinagio di tiletta falsa, di colori acquamarina
34 Uno paviglıuni, con sua cultra di velo di Napoli
35 Uno paro di pendagli di perni finti ingastati in oro, di peso di tri quarti, e trenta cocci
36 Un cascittino di cristallo, con suoi legaturi di oro, di peso di una unza, una quata et menza
37 Una rusetta di coralli con matriperni
38 Un pomettino di argento supra indorato, di peso di una quarta, et menza
39 Uno bagnuletto di ebano alionato [...] piedi et mappi di argento
40 Un cannistro grandi di argento intagliato, di peso di libre 4 et unzi due
41 Quattro sotto coppi usati di argento di peso di libre sei, et onze nove
42 Un lamperi da Cappella d'argento intagliato di peso di libre due, et onze due
43 Un fonte d'acqua benedetta d'argento per capizzo con suo crocifisso, di peso di libra una, et onze undici
44 Una inguantera di argento indorata, et intagliata, di peso onze dieci
45 Dui piatti verdi d'argento di peso di libre dieci
46 Un altro fonti d'acqua benedetta d'argento piccolo di peso di onze cinque
47 Tre para di candelieri d'argento, con dui para di meccalumi d'argento, di peso di libre 13 et onze due
48 Un bacile di tavolo grande con suo buccero d'argento, tutti dorati, di peso libre otto, et onze nove
49 Trenta piattigli di argento, di peso libre 45
50 Dudici piatti mezzani, et ordinarij d'argento, di peso di libre 27 et onze dui
51 Due bozze di argento per rinfrescare, di peso di libre sei, et onze tre
52 Dodici [...] e dudici cucchiarelli d'argento, alcune spezzate, di peso di libre quattro, et onze quattro
53 Un tenelletto di argento di peso libre 4 et onze tre
54 Un tianetto di argento, di peso libra una
55 Una candila da oglio, d'argento, di peso di libre due
56 Un scalfa vivande d'argento di peso di libre due et onze undici
57 Un cucchiarone di argento di peso di unzi sei, et quarto uno
58 Due ciotole d'argento, di peso di libra una et onza una
59 Dui gotti di argento indorato di peso di libra una et menza
Un bacile di argento da camera, con suo buccero di argento, di peso di libre 8 et onze una
Dui piatti di tavola d'acqua in mano, con perfili di oro et cum buccero d'argento, di peso libre 9 et onze 10
Una confittera d'argento, con suo coperchio d'argento, di peso libre due et onza una
Un sicchetto d'argento, di peso onze cinque, et quarti tre
Due cupetti di argento per brodo di peso di libra una, et onze due
Una salera d'argento indorata, di peso di libra una, onze due, et una quarta
Due pumetti di argento dorati per acque d'oduri, di peso di libra una, et onze dui
Una ciotula grande di argento con crocchiule, di peso di onze otto, et menza
Una scatula d'argento di peso di onze otto
Un quatro in tavola dello sposalizio di Santa Caterina, con guarnizione d'ebano all'intorno
Un altro quatro in tavola della dicesa di Croce di nostro Signore Gesù, con guarnizioni di ebano
Un altro quatro in tela, di San Giovanni Evangelista, con cornice negra
Due altri quatri pari, uno di S. Pietro, et uno di S. Paolo in tela con la cornice negra
Un quatro di un ballo di puttini, con cornice negra
Un quatro di S. Agata con guarnizione negra
Un quatro di Giuditta, con guarnizione negra
Un quatro di Coviello, con guarnizione negra
Un ritratto del quondam sig. Desiderio, di mano di Antonio Vandich, con guarnizione negra
Un quatro di nostra Signora in tavola con guarnizione di noce
Un quatro di nostro Gesù morto con guarnazione dorata
Un quatretto di S. Carlo in pietra con guarnizione di ebano
Un quatro di S. Rosalia in gloria, di mano di Antonio Vandich, con guarnizione negra
Un quatro di esposizione in croce, di mano dello stesso, con guarnizione come sopra
Un quatro di una testa che badiglia, di mano dello stesso Vandich, con guarnizione nigra et dorata
Un quatro della disputa di Cristo,

con guarnazione negra
Un quatro di Sant'Antonino con guarnazione negra
Un quatro di un bagno di Ninfe, sopra pietra, di mano del Cambiaso con guarnizione negra
Un quatro del ritratto di Amilcare Anguisciola, di mano della Signora Domina Sofonisba sua figlia
Un quatro di S. Germano, in tavola con guarnazione negra
Una cultra di raso giallo per letto incottonata
Una buffetta d'ebano perfilata d'avolio
Un'altra buffetta d'ebano lavorata d'avolio et matriperla
Una buffettina d'ebano et avolio
Un crocifisso d'avolio, con croce d'ebano
Un scrittoio fatto a contatore d'ebano, et avolio
Una scrivania d'ebano allionato, con i suoi pedi, calamaro et rinaloro d'argento
Dudici seggi grandi di alacca rossa, con frinzo di seta
Sei seggi piccoli d'alacca dorati con frinze
Un tappito grande di tavola menato
Diversi libri di poesia, et istoria, grandi et piccoli, da 60 in circa
Due baulli di vacchetta russa grandi uguali usati
Un ferriolo et un rubuni di sassonia nigri
Un vostito di perp[...] cappellano, cum calzuni, e casacca, e ferriolo, cum fodra di vellutino, et suo gippone del medesimo vellutino, colle calzette di seta arancina
Un altro vestito di panno sassoniano verduni a farriolo, foderato di velluto piano rosato, et gipponi del medesimo velluto guarnuto d'oro, con pollaino del medesimo panno, verdone, et le calzette di seta usata
Un ferriolo di tabì acqua marino [...] con fodera di mezzo vellutino acqua marino bianco, e gialno, con vestito della medesima forma
Calzuni o gipponi di velluto negro
Un ferriolo di burattino [...] nigro, infoderato di terzanello undiato picato
Un coiretto di danto, con passamano d'oro
Un coiretto di pelle di Roma, con passamani d'oro, foderato di trezzanello acqua marina
Un paio di manichi di velluto negro ad orli di raso negri
Un paro di calzuni di rasetto per sutta di dui culuri
Un ferriolo di bajetta negra, foderato di felba negra
Un altro ferriolo di panno di ventiquattrino, di colore scuro, con felba acquamarina
Un cammiciolo di damasco lionato, con buttuni di ramo dorati
Una spata, et un pugnali argentati, cum suo pendenti, et cinturino
Un'altra spata, et pugnali intagliati et indorati, con suo centurino, et pendenti di canettiglio
Due scupettini a rota alla bresciana
Due caxettini piccoli uguali coperti di vacchetta rossa
Un paviglione di panno torchino con sua coperta
Due scrittorielli di ebano, intagliati di avolio, simili ambidui uguali
Sei pezzi di panni di razza, menati di verdure
Un saimbarco di panno turchino, foderato di bajetta verde, usati
Un paviglione di filo a un dente, listato di rete lavorato, con una frinza attorno

* Transcribed in Di Giovanni 1889.

Appendix 3

Contract for the *Madonna of the Rosary* for the Oratorio del SS. Rosario at San Domenico, 22 August 1625. Archivio di Stato, Palermo, Not. Vincenzo Sarago, stanza II, vol. 1862, ff. 419r–420r*

Die 22 mensis Aug[us]ti 8 Ind. 1625

Antonius Vandich flander mihi not[a]rio cog[ni]tus p[raese]ns coram nobis sponte promisit, seq[ue] solemniter oblig[av]it,
et obligat Francisco Barrales gubernatori Petro Martinelli,
& Io[anni] Jacobo Calderaro coniunctis ven[erabilis] sodalitatis sancta Mariae sacratissimi rosarij sancti Dom[ini]ci sub titulo delli sacchi, nec non & Antonio della torre uni ex sodalibus ipsius sodalitatis mihi not[ario] et cog[nit]is p[raese]ntibus et stipulantibus nom[in]e eiusdem sodalitatis depingere proprijs ipsius Antonij sumptibus et exp[ens]is iconam diva Maria sacratissii rosarij modo, forma, & cum conditionibus quibus infra nimirum Depingere nella città di Napoli, o in altro luogo d'Italia un quatro in tela d'altezza di palmi quindeci, e di larghezza di palmi dieci, e tre quarti con l'imagine di nostra signora del Rosario, san Domenico, san Vicenzo, santa Caterina di Siena, santa Rosolea, santa Christina, Nimfa, Oliva, et Agata conforme al disegno, che d[ett]i gover[nato]re, congiunti, e d[ett]o fr[at]ello eligeranno: con che esso Antonio sia tenuto fare tre disegni coloriti, e quelli inviare qua in Palermo, o consegnarli in Napoli, o in altro luogo al commissionaro di d[ett]o di Barrales, o di d[ett]o della torre ad effetto di mandarlo qua alle sud[dett]e persone a d[ett]o nome. le quali, visti li detti tre disegni, habiano da dechiarare sopra quale vorranno che si faccia d[ett]o quatro. e fatta la dechiaratione di d[ett]o disegno, che eligeranno, habiano quello da signare di loro proprio nome, & inviarlo a d[ett]o Antonio. Il quale Antonio, havuto il disegno predetto, sia tenuto cominciare, seguitare e finire il detto quatro bene, diligente, e magistrevolmente con colori fini e di buona conditione, et in particolare che il colore torchino per il manto della Madonna, et altre cose di d[ett]o quatro sia oltra marino fino fra termine di mesi sei da contarsi d'hoggi innanti. Con questo però che, finito, e spedito che sarrà il detto quatro s'habia da fare rivedere per doi esperti, che eligeranno li commissionati di d[ett]o di Barrale, e d[ett]o della torre. & essendosi trovato il d[ett]o quatro conforme al disegno, e di piu bene, diligente, e magistrevolmente fatto, ben disegnato, e ben colorito con le sue ombre, e chiari, conforme l'arte richiede, e delle condizioni dette di sopra, esso Antonio habia quello da consignare in detta città di Napoli, o in altro luogo, dove si trovera ad uno delli commissionati di detti di Barrales, e la torre, e non altrimente, ne in altro modo.

Alias &c.

Et hoc pro mercede, & manupretio ducatorum biscentorum sexaginta monete neapolitane currentis quam quidem mercedem,
& manupretium prenominate persone nom[inat]e ipsius sodalitatis dare, ac realiter, et cum effectu solvere promiserunt, seque solemniter obligaverunt, et obligant eidem Antonio p[rese]nti, et stip[ulan]ti vel persone pro eo legitime aut in ditta c[ivita]te Neapoli, aut eius valorem in alio quovis loco ubi consignatio d[icte]e icone fiet, facta prius consignatione pred[ict]a statim,
& excontinenti. Omnibus quidem oppositionibus, omnibusque exceptionibus iuris, et facti remotis poenitus, & expresse renunciantis.

Coeterum ipse Antonij ad instantiam predictarum personarum p[raese]ntium, & stipulantium n[omin]e dicte sodalitatis dixit, et confessus est se ab eisdem habuisse, et recepisse telam, super qua d[ict]a icona depingi debet, impressam pro effectu predicto. Idque vero gratis.
R.ns exceptionis &c.
Quae omnia &c. pro.nt rata habere &c. in omnem eventum &c. In pace et de plano &c.

Sub hyp[ote]ca et obligatione omnium, & singulorum bonorum eorum mob. & stab. &c. cum refectione damnorum, interesse, et expensarum litis, et ex[tr]a, etiam viaticarum &c. Et fiat ritus, et executio in persona, et bonis d[ict]i Antonij, & in bonis tantum d[ict]e sodalitatis, et variari possit &c. Adversus quem ritum, ex.onem, formam p[raese]ntis contractis, & extremorum verificationem non possint se opp.re &c. Quin prius adimpleatur tenor, et forma p[raese]ntis contractus, et pignora &c. Renuntiantes &c.

Et specialiter cum iuramento beneficio [...] moratoria, guidatici, supersessorie quinquennalis dilationis cessionis bonorum &c. Nec non beneficio restitutionis in integrum &c.

Et pred.a att.res &c.
Iuraverunt &c.
Testes not. Cesar Lametta, Nicolaus Freirone, Jiuliu Scigliano, Dominicus Lanfrucco, et Petrus Darrigo

* Another copy of the contract is in ASP, Not. Vincenzo Sarago, stanza II, vol. 1870, ff. 562r–563v.

Bibliography

Manuscripts

Auria (no date)
G.F. Auria, *Croniche varie di Sicilia, ed altre cose notabili trascritte dall'Auria*, Biblioteca Comunale, Palermo, Ms. Qq E55

Britton 1813
J. Britton, *A Brief Catalogue of Pictures, Late the Property of Sir Francis Bourgeois…* Ms. London, Dulwich College Archive, London 1813

Maya (no date)
C. Maya, *Relazione di quello che fece la città di Palermo per il male contagioso di peste, che afflisse detta città da' 7 maggio 1624 sino a 6 giugno 1626, giorno in cui si diede l'ultima volta l'universal pratica*, Biblioteca Comunale, Palermo, Ms. Qq C 33

Raccolta sulla peste
Raccolta di originali scritture e stampe sulla peste di Palermo degli anni 1624 e 1625, oltre alcune di altre pestilenze, Biblioteca Comunale, Palermo, Ms. Qq H 59

Printed sources

Abbate 1990
V. Abbate, 'Quadrerie e collezionisti palermitani del Seicento', in *Pittori del Seicento a Palazzo Abatellis*, exhibition catalogue, V. Abbate ed., Palermo 1990, pp. 13–57

Abbate 1991
V. Abbate, 'Il '600: Santa Rosalia nella rappresentazione pittorica', in A. Gerbino ed., *La Rosa dell'Ercta*, Palermo 1991, pp. 91–108

Abbate 1999a
V. Abbate, 'La città aperta. Pittura e società a Palermo tra Cinque e Seicento', in *Porto di mare 1570–1670. Pittori e pittura a Palermo tra memoria e recupero*, exhibition catalogue, V. Abbate ed., Palermo 1999, pp. 11–56

Abbate 1999b
V. Abbate, 'La stagione del grande collezionismo', in *Porto di mare 1570–1670. Pittori e pittura a Palermo tra memoria e recupero*, exhibition catalogue, V. Abbate ed., Palermo 1999, pp. 107–40

Abbate 2001
F. Abbate, *Storia dell'arte nell'Italia meridionale*, Rome 2001

Abbate 2004
V. Abbate, 'Van Dyck a Palermo', in *Anton van Dyck. Riflessi italiani*, exhibition catalogue, M.G. Bernardini ed., Milan 2004, pp. 69–81

Abbate 2011
V. Abbate, *La grande stagione del collezionismo. Mecenati, accademie e mercato dell'arte in Sicilia tra Cinque e Seicento*, Palermo 2011

Adriani 1940
G. Adriani, *Anton van Dyck. Italienisches Skizzenbuch*, Vienna 1940

Ainsworth 1982
M. Ainsworth *et al.*, *Art and Autoradiography: Insights into the Genesis of Paintings by Rembrandt, Van Dyck and Vermeer*, New York 1982

Antwerp 1899
Van Dijck Tentoonstelling, exhibition catalogue, Antwerp 1899

Ascenso 1692
F. Ascenso, *La mano tutta mano di S. Rosalia, vergine palermitana: panegirico sacro*, Messina 1692

Astrua and Spantigati 2000
P. Astrua and C.E. Spantigati, *Galleria Sabauda. Short Guide*, Turin 2000

Baetjer 2004
K. Baetjer, 'Buying Pictures for New York: The Founding Purchase of 1871', *Metropolitan Museum Journal* 39 (2004), pp. 161–245

Bailey 2005
G.A. Bailey, 'Anthony Van Dyck, the Cult of Saint Rosalie, and the 1624 Plague in Palermo', in *Hope and Healing. Painting in Italy in a Time of Plague 1500–1800*, exhibition catalogue, G.A. Bailey, P.M. Jones, F. Mormando and T.W. Worcester eds., Worcester 2005, pp. 118–36

Baldass 1957
L. Baldass, 'Some Notes on the Development of Van Dyck's Portrait Style', *Gazette des Beaux-Arts* 50 (1957), pp. 251–70

Barnes 1986
S.J. Barnes, *Van Dyck in Italy: 1621–1628*, Ph.D. Thesis, New York University, 1986

Barnes, De Poorter, Millar, Vey 2004
S.J. Barnes, N. De Poorter, O. Millar and H. Vey, *Van Dyck. A Complete Catalogue of the Paintings*, New Haven and London 2004

Barnes and Wheelock 1994
S.J. Barnes and A.K. Wheelock eds., *Van Dyck 350. Studies in the History of Art 46*, Washington 1994

Baudi di Vesme 1885
A. Baudi di Vesme, *Van Dyck peintre de portraits des princes de Savoie*, Turin 1885

Bauman and Liedtke 1992
G.C. Bauman and W.A. Liedtke, *Flemish Paintings in America. A Survey of Early Netherlandish and Flemish paintings in the Public Collections of North America*, Antwerp 1992

Baumstark 1980
R. Baumstark, *Masterpieces from the Collection of the Princes of Liechtenstein*, New York 1980

Bellori 2005
G.P. Bellori, *The Lives of the Modern Painters, Sculptors and Architects*, translated by A. Sedgwick Wohl, Cambridge 2005

Bellori 2009
G.P. Bellori, *Le vite de' pittori, scultori e architetti moderni*, Rome 1672, E. Borea ed., Turin 2009

Beresford 1998
R. Beresford, *Dulwich Picture Gallery. Complete Illustrated Catalogue*, London 1998

Bermejo 1820
D. Bermejo, *Descripción artística del Real Monasterio de San Lorenzo del Escorial y sus preciosidades después de la invasion de los franceses*, Madrid 1820

Bethencourt 1992
F. Bethencourt, 'The *Auto da Fé*: Ritual and Imagery', *Journal of the Warburg and Courtauld Institutes* 55 (1992), pp. 155–68

Blake 1999
R. Blake, *Anthony van Dyck. A Life 1599–1641*, London 1999

Blunt 1958
A. Blunt, 'Poussin Studies VII: Poussins in Neapolitan and Sicilian Collections', *The Burlington Magazine* 100 (1958), pp. 76–86

Boccia and Coelho 1967
L.G. Boccia and E.T. Coelho, *L'arte dell'armatura in Italia*, Milan 1967

Boccia and Godoy 1987
L.G. Boccia and J.A. Godoy, 'La armadura del Príncipe Emanuele Filiberto de Saboya (1588–1624)', *Reales Sitios* 24 (1987), pp. 57–68

Bode 1889
W. von Bode, 'Anton van Dyck (in der Liechtenstein Galerie)', *Die Graphischen Künste* 12 (1889), pp. 39–52

Bolten and Folmer-von Oven 1989
J. Bolten and A.T. Folmer-von Oven, *Catalogue of Drawings [of a Private Collection]*, Hilversum 1989

Bottineau 1956
Y. Bottineau, 'L'Alcázar de Madrid et l'inventaire de 1686. Aspects de la cour d'Espagne au XVIIe Siècle', *Bulletin Hispanique* 58 (1956), pp. 421–52

Bottineau 1958
Y. Bottineau, 'L'Alcázar de Madrid et l'inventaire de 1686. Aspects de la cour d'Espagne au XVIIe siècle', *Bulletin His-*

panique 60 (1958), pp. 30–61, 145–79, 289–326, 450–83

Brady 1839
J.H. Brady, *The Visitor's Guide to Knole*, London 1839

Brandus 1928
E. Brandus, 'La Collection des Tableaux Anciens de M. Jules S. Bache, aNew-York', *La Renaissance* 11 (1928), pp. 192–94

Bridgman 1817
J. Bridgman, *An Historical and Topographical Sketch of Knole*, London 1817

Briggs 1996
R. Briggs, *Witches and Neighbours: the Social and Cultural Context of European Witchcraft*, London 1996

Brigstocke 1982
H. Brigstocke, *William Buchanan and the 19th-century Art Trade*, London 1982

Brown 1982
C. Brown, *Van Dyck*, New York 1982

Brown and Ramsay 1990
C. Brown and N. Ramsay, 'Van Dyck's Collection: Some New Documents', *The Burlington Magazine* 132 (1990), pp. 704–09

Buchanan 1824
W. Buchanan, *Memoirs of Painting*, London 1824

Cabibbo 2004
S. Cabibbo, *Santa Rosalia tra terra e cielo. Storia, rituali, linguaggi di un culto barocco*, Palermo 2004

Catalogo 1952
Museo del Prado. Catalogo de las Pinturas, Madrid 1952

Catalogue 1872
Catalogue of the Pictures in the Metropolitan Museum of Art, New York 1872

Churchill 1908
S.J.A. Churchill, 'Sir Anthony van Dyck's Visit to Sicily About 1624', *The Burlington Magazine* 14 (1908), pp. 239–40

Cifani and Monetti 1990
A. Cifani and F. Monetti, *Arte e artisti nel Piemonte del '600. Nuove scoperte e nuovi orientamenti*, Cavallermaggiore 1990

Collura 1977
P. Collura, *Santa Rosalia nella storia e nell'arte*, Palermo 1977

Collura 1994
P. Collura, 'La vita di Santa Rosalia', in M.C. Di Natale ed., *S. Rosaliae Patriae Servatrici*, Palermo 1994, pp. 9–10

Contino and Mantia 1998
A. Contino and S. Mantia, *Vincenzo La Barbera architetto e pittore termitano*, Bagheria 1998

Costello 1950
J. Costello, 'The twelve pictures "ordered by Velasquez" and the trial of Valguarnera', *Journal of the Warburg and Courtauld Institutes* 13 (1950), pp. 237–84

Cremona, Vienna and Washington 1994
Sofonisba Anguissola e le sue sorelle, exhibition catalogue, M. Gregori ed., Cremona, Vienna and Washington 1994

Cust 1900
L. Cust, *Anthony van Dyck: An Historical Study of His Life and Works*, London 1900

Cust 1902
L. Cust, *A Description of the Sketch-book by Sir Anthony van Dyck used by him in Italy, 1621–1627, and preserved in the Collection of the Duke of Devonshire, K.G., at Chatsworth*, London 1902

Cust 1911
L. Cust, *Van Dyck: A Further Study*, London 1911

De Andrés 1971
G. de Andrés, 'Relacíon anónima del siglo XVII sobre los cuadros del Escorial', *Archivio Español de Arte* 173 (1971), pp. 54–55

De Frutos 2009
L. de Frutos, *El Templo de la Fama. Alegoría del Marqués del Carpio*, Madrid 2009

De Gennaro 2003
R. De Gennaro, *Per il collezionismo del Seicento in Sicilia: L'*Inventario *di Antonio Ruffo Principe della Scaletta*, Pisa 2003

De los Santos 1667
F. de los Santos, *Descripción del Real Monasterio de San Lorenzo del Escorial*, Madrid 1667

De Seta 2002
C. de Seta, *Palermo: Città d'arte*, Palermo 2002

Di Giovanni 1889
V. Di Giovanni, 'I Paruta in Palermo e nella signoria del Castello di Sala di Madonna Alvira, indi Sala di Paruta', *Archivio Storico Siciliano* 14 (1889), pp. 269–92

Di Natale 1994
M.C. Di Natale ed., *S. Rosaliae Patriae Servatrici*, Palermo 1994

Di Natale 1998
M.C. Di Natale, *Capolavori del Museo Diocesano 'ex sacris imaginibus magnum fructum'*, Palermo 1998

Di Natale 2006
M.C. Di Natale, *Il Museo Diocesano di Palermo*, Palermo 2006

Du Gué Trapier 1957
E. Du Gué Trapier, 'The School of Madrid and Van Dyck', *The Burlington Magazine* 99 (1957), pp. 265–73

Egger 1942
H. Egger, 'Anton Van Dyck: Italienisches Skizzenbuch im Herbst 1622. Beiträge zur Kritik des Chatsworther Skizzenbuches', *Die Graphischen Künste* 7 (1942), pp. 29–39

Ekserdjian 2000
D. Ekserdjian, 'Van Dyck and the Old Masters. A Drawing and its Sources', *Apollo* 151 (2000), pp. 46–48

Evelyn 1850
J. Evelyn, *Diary and Correspondence of John Evelyn*, W. Bray ed., London 1850

Failla 2003
M.B. Failla, 'Il principe Emanuele Filiberto di Savoia. Collezioni e committenze tra ducato sabaudo, corte spagnola e viceregno di Sicilia', in M.B. Failla and C. Goria eds., *Committenti d'età barocca. Le collezioni del principe Emanuele Filiberto di Savoia a Palermo e la decorazione di Palazzo Taffini d'Acceglio a Savigliano*, Turin 2003, pp. 13–112

Fanti 1767
V. Fanti, *Descrizzione completa di tutto ciò che ritrovasi nella galleria di pittura e scultura di Sua Altezza Giuseppe Wenceslao del S.R.I. Principe Regnante della casa di Liechtenstein*, Vienna 1767

Filipczak 1989
Z.Z. Filipczak, 'Van Dyck's Life of St Rosalie', *The Burlington Magazine* 131 (1989), pp. 693–98

Gabrielli 1971
N. Gabrielli, *Galleria Sabauda. Maestri Italiani*, Turin 1971

Gaya Nuño 1964
J.A. Gaya Nuño, *Pintura europea perdida por España. De Van Eyck a Tiépolo*, Madrid 1964

Genoa 1955
100 Opere di Van Dyck, exhibition catalogue, C. Marcenaro *et al.*, Genoa 1955

Genoa 1997
Van Dyck a Genova. Grande pittura e collezionismo, exhibition catalogue, S.J. Barnes, P. Boccardo, C. Di Fabio and L. Tagliaferro eds., Genoa 1997

Gerbino 1991
A. Gerbino ed., *La Rosa dell'Ercta*, Palermo 1991

Giltaij 1999
J. Giltaij, *Ruffo en Rembrandt. Over een Siciliaanse verzamelaar in de zeventiende*

eeuw die drie schilderijen bij Rembrandt bestelde, Zutphen 1999

Giordano 1997
R.C. Giordano ed., *Originale delli testimonij di Santa Rosalia*, Palermo 1997

Giuditta 1671
La giuditta palermitana, ovvero la Vergine S. Rosalia, triomfatrice d'Oloferne, cioé la Peste, Palermo 1671

Glück 1925
G. Glück, *The Early Work of Van Dyck*, Vienna 1925

Glück 1931
G. Glück, *Van Dyck. Des Meisters Gemälde*, Stuttgart and Berlin 1931

Glück 1934
G. Glück, 'Self-Portraits by Van Dyck and Jordaens', *The Burlington Magazine* 65 (1934), pp. 195–201

Godoy 1987
J.A. Godoy, 'Notes sur quelques armures du "Maestro dal Castello"', *Genava*, 35 (1987), pp. 11–34

Guiffrey 1882
J. Guiffrey, *Antoine van Dyck: sa vie et son œuvre*, Paris 1882

Held 1965
J.S. Held, *Museo de Arte de Ponce. Catalogue. I. Paintings of the European and American Schools*, Ponce 1965

Held 1984
J.S. Held, *Museo de Arte de Ponce. Fundación Luis A. Ferré. Catalogue. Paintings and Sculpture of the European and American Schools*, Ponce 1984

Hipp 2007
E. Hipp, 'Poussin's *The Plague at Ashdod*. A Work of Art in Multiple Contexts', in F. Mormando and T. Worcester eds., *Piety and Plague. From Byzantium to the Baroque*, Kirksville, Missouri 2007, pp. 177–223

Houston 1968
A Young Teaching Collection, exhibition catalogue, Houston 1968

Jaffé 2001
D. Jaffé, 'New Thoughts on Van Dyck's Italian Sketchbook', *The Burlington Magazine* 143 (2001), pp. 614–24

Jaffé 2002
M. Jaffé, *The Devonshire Collection of Northern European Drawings*, 5 vols., Turin 2002

James 1956
H. James, *The Painter's Eye. Notes and Essays on the Pictorial Arts*, London 1956

Jameson 1842
A. Jameson, *Handbook to the Public Galleries of Art in and near London*, London 1842

Jubinal and Sensi 1839
A. Jubinal and G. Sensi, *La Armería Real ou collection des principales pièces de la galerie d'armes anciennes de Madrid*, Paris 1839

Kauffmann 1982
M.C. Kauffmann, *Catalogue of Paintings in the Wellington Museum*, London 1982

Kauffmann and Jenkins 2009
M.C. Kauffmann and S. Jenkins, *Catalogue of Paintings in the Wellington Museum, Apsley House*, London 2009

LaRocca 2000
D.J. LaRocca, 'A Notable Group of Late Sixteenth-Century Etched Italian Armour', *The Arms & Armour Society* 16 (2000), pp. 181–97

Larsen 1980a
E. Larsen, *L'opera completa di Van Dyck 1613–1626*, Milan 1980

Larsen 1980b
E. Larsen, *L'opera completa di Van Dyck 1626–1641*, Milan 1980

Larsen 1988
E. Larsen, *The Paintings of Anthony van Dyck*, Freren 1988

Liechtenstein 1780
Description des tableaux et des pieces de sculpture que renferme la gallerie de son altesse François Joseph, chef et Prince regnant de la maison de Liechtenstein, Vienna 1780

Liedtke 1984a
W.A. Liedtke, *Flemish Paintings in The Metropolitan Museum of Art*, New York 1984

Liedtke 1984b
W.A. Liedtke, *Anthony van Dyck, The Metropolitan Museum of Art Bulletin XLII*, New York 1984

Liedtke 1989
W. Liedtke, 'Dutch and Flemish Paintings from the Hermitage: Some notes to an exhibition catalogue, with special attention to Rembrandt, Van Dyck and Jordaens', *Oud Holland* 103 (1989), pp. 154–68

Litta 1872
P. Litta, *Famiglie celebri italiane*, vol. 10, Milan 1872

Little 1995
N.J. Little, 'Van Dyck's "Saint John in the Wilderness"', *IFAR Reports* 16 (1995), pp. 1–5

London 1900
Exhibition of the Works by Van Dyck 1599–1641, exhibition catalogue, London 1900

London 1982
Van Dyck in England, exhibition catalogue, O. Millar ed., London 1982

London 1995a
Death, Passion and Politics. Van Dyck's Portraits of Venetia Stanley and George Digby, exhibition catalogue, A. Sumner ed., London 1995

London 1995b
In Trust for the Nation. Paintings from National Trust Houses, A. Laing ed., London 1995

London 1999a
Van Dyck 1599–1641, exhibition catalogue, C. Brown and H. Vlieghe eds., London 1999

London 1999b
Van Dyck at the Wallace Collection, exhibition catalogue, J. Hedley ed., London 1999

London 1999c
The Light of Nature. Landscape Drawing and Watercolours by Van Dyck and his Contemporaries, exhibition catalogue, M. Royalton-Kisch ed., London 1999

London 2009
Van Dyck and Britain, exhibition catalogue, K. Hearn ed., London 2009

Maclarnon 1990
K. Maclarnon, 'William Bankes and his Collection of Spanish Paintings at Kingston Lacy', *Burlington Magazine* 132 (1990), pp. 114–25

Madrid 2010
El arte del poder. La Real Armería y el retrato de corte, exhibition catalogue, A. Soler del Campo ed., Madrid 2010

Madrid and Bilbao 1999
Obras Maestras de la Dulwich Picture Gallery, exhibition catalogue, C. Giménez ed., Madrid and Bilbao 1999

Mariette 1851
P.-J. Mariette, *Abecedario de P.-J. Mariette et autres notes inédites de cet auteur sur les arts et les Artistes*, Paris 1851

Martínez del Romero 1849
A. Martínez del Romero, *Catálogo de la Real Armería*, Madrid 1849

Matranga 1908
C. Matranga, 'Dipinti di Antonio van Dijck e della sua scuola nel Museo Nazionale di Palermo', *Bollettino d'Arte* 2 (1908), pp. 11–18

Mazzola 1997
M.G. Mazzola, 'Matthias Stomer a Palermo: alcuni inediti per la sua biografia', *Storia dell'Arte* 89 (1997), pp. 67–73

McGrath 2001
E. McGrath, '"Una striga in Palermo". A Sicilian Document from the Italian Sketchbook', in H. Vlieghe ed., *Van Dyck 1599–1999. Conjectures and Refutations*, Turnhout 2001, pp. 43–51

Mele 2003
G. Mele, *Santa Rosalia: Storia e leggenda della patrona di Palermo*, Palermo 2003

Meli 1878
G. Meli, 'Documenti relativi a un quadro dell'altar maggiore dell'Oratorio della Compagnia del Rosario di S. Domenico', *Archivio Storico Siciliano* 3 (1878), p. 210

Mendola 1999a
G. Mendola, 'Dallo Zoppo di Gangi a Pietro Novelli. Nuove acquisizioni documentarie', in *Porto di mare 1570–1670. Pittori e pittura a Palermo tra memoria e recupero*, exhibition catalogue, V. Abbate ed., Palermo 1999, pp. 57–87

Mendola 1999b
G. Mendola, 'Un approdo sicuro. Nuovi documenti per Van Dyck e Gerardi a Palermo', in *Porto di mare 1570–1670. Pittori e pittura a Palermo tra memoria e recupero*, exhibition catalogue, V. Abbate ed., Palermo 1999, pp. 88–106

Mendola 1999c
G. Mendola, 'Van Dyck in Sicily', in *Van Dyck 1599–1641*, exhibition catalogue, C. Brown and H. Vlieghe eds., London 1999, pp. 58–63

Messana 2007
M.S. Messana, *Inquisitori, negromanti e streghe nella Sicilia moderna (1500–1782)*, Palermo 2007

Milan 2004
Anton van Dyck. Riflessi italiani, exhibition catalogue, M.G. Bernardini ed., Milan 2004

Millar 1969
O. Millar, 'Notes on Three Pictures by Van Dyck', *The Burlington Magazine* 111 (1969), pp. 414–18

Millar 1997
O. Millar, 'Review of Van Dyck in

Genoa', *The Burlington Magazine* 139 (1997), pp. 500–04

Moir 1994
A. Moir, *Anthony van Dyck*, New York 1994

Montebello 1963
G.P. de Montebello, 'Van Dyck, Painter of the Counter Reformation', *Metropolitan Museum of Art Bulletin* 22 (1963), pp. 133–42

Mormando and Worcester 2007
F. Mormando and T. Worcester eds., *Piety and Plague. From Byzantium to the Baroque*, Kirksville, Missouri 2007

Morreale 1990
A. Morreale, 'Libri, quadri e "artificiose machine". L'inventario di Don Marco Gezio cappellano della Cattedrale di Palermo (1658)', in *Annali della Facoltà di Lettere e Filosofia dell'Università di Palermo* (1990)

Morreale 1999
A. Morreale, 'Palermo: la cultura del Seicento', in *Porto di mare 1570–1670. Pittori e pittura a Palermo tra memoria e recupero*, exhibition catalogue, V. Abbate ed., Palermo 1999, pp. 141–46

Münster 1998
1648. War and Peace in Europe, exhibition catalogue, Münster 1998

Murray 1980
P. Murray, *Dulwich Picture Gallery. A Catalogue*, London 1980

Naples 2007
Omaggio a Capodimonte: da Caravaggio a Picasso, exhibition catalogue, N. Spinosa ed., Museo di Capodimonte, Naples 2007

Negri Arnoldi 1984
F. Negri Arnoldi, 'Pittori fiamminghi in Sicilia tra Rubens e Caravaggio', *Prospettiva* 39 (1984), pp. 60–67

New York 1985
Liechtenstein: The Princely Collections, exhibition catalogue, R. Baumstark *et al.*, New York 1985

New York and Fort Worth 1991
The Drawings of Anthony van Dyck, exhibition catalogue, C. Brown ed., New York and Fort Worth 1991

Ottawa 1980
The Young Van Dyck, exhibition catalogue, A. McNairn ed., Ottawa 1980

Palazzotto 2003
P. Palazzotto, *Da Santa Rosalia a Santa Rosalia. Opere d'arte restaurate del Museo Diocesano di Palermo dal XVII al XIX secolo*, Palermo 2003

Palazzotto and Scordato 2002
P. Palazzotto and C. Scordato, *L'Oratorio del Rosario in San Domenico*, Palermo 2002

Palermo 1990a
Pittori del Seicento a Palazzo Abatellis, exhibition catalogue, V. Abbate ed., Palermo 1990

Palermo 1990b
Pietro Novelli e il suo ambiente, exhibition catalogue, M. Calvesi *et al.*, Palermo 1990

Palermo 1999
Porto di mare 1570–1670. Pittori e pittura a Palermo tra memoria e recupero, exhibition catalogue, V. Abbate ed., Palermo 1999

Paris 2008
Antoon van Dyck. Portraits, exhibition catalogue, A. Merle du Bourg ed., Paris 2008

Patricolo 2006
R. Patricolo, *San Giorgio dei Genovesi. Le fabbriche, le stirpi, i simboli, le epigrafi*, Palermo 2006

Phoenix, Memphis and Nashville 2008
Masterpieces of European Painting from Museo de Arte de Ponce, exhibition catalogue, C. Hartup and R. Aste eds., Phoenix, Memphis and Nashville 2008

Pinto and Di Macco 1991
S. Pinto and M. Di Macco, *Guide brevi della Galleria Sabauda. Secondo settore. Collezioni dinastiche: da Vittorio Amedeo I a Vittorio Amedeo II 1630–1730*, Turin 1991

Ponz 1776
A. Ponz, *Viage de España*, vol. 5–6, Madrid 1776

Princeton 1979
Van Dyck as Religious Artist, exhibition catalogue, J.R. Martin and G. Feigenbaum eds., Princeton 1979

Prohaska 1996
W. Prohaska, 'I rapporti di Ribera con la pittura fiamminga in area mediterranea: il caso Van Dyck', *Ricerche sul '600 napoletano. Scritti in memoria di Raffaello Causa* (1996), pp. 210–22

Reina 2005
G. Reina, *L'Eremo della Quisquina*, Agrigento 2005

Renda 2003
F. Renda, *Storia della Sicilia dalle origini ai giorni nostri*, Palermo 2003

Richter and Sparkes 1880
J.P. Richter and J.C.L. Sparkes eds., *Catalogue of the Pictures in the Dulwich College Gallery with Biographical Notices of the Painters*, London 1880

Roethlisberger 2002
M. Roethlisberger *et al.*, *100 Masterpieces. Museo de Arte de Ponce*, Ponce 2002

Rome 1994
Roma 1630. Il trionfo del pennello, exhibition catalogue, O. Bonfait ed., Rome 1994

Rose 1983
I. Rose, *Manuel Godoy, Patron de las artes y Collecionista*, Madrid 1983

Rotondi Terminiello 1980
G. Rotondi Terminiello *et al.*, *Genova e i Genovesi a Palermo. Atti delle manifestazioni culturali tenutesi a Genova, 13 dicembre 1978 / 13 gennaio 1979*, Genoa 1980

Ruffo 1916
V. Ruffo, 'Galleria Ruffo nel secolo XVII in Messina (con lettere di pittori ed altri documenti inediti)', *Bollettino d'Arte* 10 (1916), pp. 21–64, 95–128, 165–92, 237–56, 284–320, 369–88

Ruffo 1919
V. Ruffo, 'La Galleria Ruffo (Appendice)', *Bollettino d'Arte* 13 (1919), pp. 43–56

Sacchi 1994
R. Sacchi, 'Tra la Sicilia e Genova: Sofonisba Anguissola Moncada e poi Lomellini', in *Sofonisba Anguissola e le sue sorelle*, exhibition catalogue, M. Gregori ed., Cremona, Vienna and Washington 1994, pp. 153–72

Salinas 1899
A. Salinas, 'Antonio Van Dijck e il suo quadro per la Compagnia del Rosario in S. Domenico', *L'Arte* 2 (1899), pp. 499–50

Sánchez Cantón 1933
F.J. Sánchez Cánton, *Fuentes literarias para la Historia del Arte Español*, Madrid 1933

Santino 1999
U. Santino, *I giorni della peste: il festino di Santa Rosalia tra mito e spettacolo*, Palermo 1999

Santoro 2003
R. Santoro, *Il festino di Santa Rosalia*, Palermo 2003

Schaeffer 1909
E. Schaeffer, *Van Dyck: des Meisters Gemälde, Klassiker der Kunst*, Stuttgart and Leipzig 1909

Sciascia 1994
L. Sciascia, 'Diamanti', in *Roma 1630. Il trionfo del pennello*, exhibition catalogue, O. Bonfait ed., Rome 1994, pp. 15–21

Servizi 2008
C. Servizi ed., *Palermo. I Tesori del quartiere della Loggia*, Milan 2008

Sitwell 1941
S. Sitwell, 'Van Dyck: An Appreciation', *The Burlington Magazine* 79 (1941), pp. 174–77

Smith 1831
J. Smith, *A Catalogue Raisonné of the Works of the Most Eminent Dutch, Flemish, and French Painters*, London 1831

Soprani 1674
R. Soprani, *Le vite de' Pittori, Scoltori et Architetti Genovesi, e de Forastieri che in Genova operarono*, Genoa 1674

Sparkes 1876
J.C.L. Sparkes, *A Descriptive Catalogue of the Pictures in the Dulwich College Gallery: with Biographical Notices of the Painters*, London 1876

Spatafora 1998
C. Spatafora, *La Compagnia del SS. Rosario in S. Domenico. L'oratorio e le sue opera d'arte*, Palermo 1998

Sterling 1939
C. Sterling, 'Van Dyck's Paintings of St. Rosalie', *The Burlington Magazine* 74 (1939), pp. 53–62

Stewart 1997
J.D. Stewart, 'Van Dyck at Genoa', *Apollo* 146 (1997), pp. 52–53

Susinno 1960
F. Susinno, *Le Vite de' Pittori Messinesi*, V. Martinelli ed., Florence 1960

Tamburini 1977
L. Tamburini, 'Carlone, Tommaso', in *Dizionario Biografico degli Italiani*, vol. 20, Rome 1977, pp. 392–94

Tietze-Conrat 1950
E. Tietze-Conrat, 'Das "Skizzenbuch" des Van Dyck als Quelle für die Tizianforschung', *Critica d'Arte* 8 (1950), pp. 425–42

Vaes 1924
M. Vaes, 'Le séjour de Van Dyck en Italie (Mi-novembre 1621 – Automne 1627)', *Bulletin de l'Institut Historique Belge de Rome* 4 (1924), pp. 163–234

Vaes 1925
M. Vaes, 'Corneille de Wael (1592–1667)', *Bulletin de l'Institut Historique Belge de Rome* 5 (1925), pp. 137–247

Vaes 1941
M. Vaes, 'Il soggiorno di Antonio van Dyck alla corte di Torino 4 dicembre – febbraio 1623', *Bollettino Storico Bibliografico Subalpino* 43 (1941), pp. 227–39

Valencia de Don Juan 1898
C.V. de Valencia de Don Juan, *Catálogo histórico-descriptivo de la Real Armería de Madrid*, Madrid 1898

Valentiner 1950
W.R. Valentiner, 'Van Dyck's Character', *Art Quarterly* 13 (1950), pp. 87–104

Van de Put 1912
A. Van de Put, '*The Prince of Oneglia* by Van Dyck', *The Burlington Magazine* 21 (1912), pp. 311–14

Van de Put 1914
A. Van de Put, 'Van Dyck's *Prince of Oneglia*', *The Burlington Magazine* 25 (1914), p. 59

Vannugli 1989
A. Vannugli, *La collezione Serra di Cassano*, Salerno 1989

Van Puyvelde 1950
L. van Puyvelde, *Van Dyck*, Brussels 1950

Venaria Reale 2007
La Reggia di Venaria e i Savoia, exhibition catalogue, E. Castelnuovo ed., Venaria Reale 2007

Venturi 1926
L. Venturi, *La Collezione Gualino*, Turin and Rome 1926

Vitella 1994
M. Vitella, 'Il primo Festino', in M.C. Di Natale ed., *S. Rosaliae Patriae Servatrici*, Palermo 1994, pp. 81–117

Vlieghe 2001
H. Vlieghe ed., *Van Dyck 1599–1999. Conjectures and Refutations*, Turnhout 2001

Waagen 1838
G.F. Waagen, *Works of Art and Artists in England*, London 1838

Waagen 1854
G.F. Waagen, *Treasures of Art in Great Britain*, London 1854

Walpole 1828
H. Walpole, *Anecdotes of Painting in England with Some Account of the Principal Artists*, London 1828

Washington 1990
Van Dyck, exhibition catalogue, S.J. Barnes and A.K. Wheelock eds., Washington 1990

Washington 1995
Sofonsiba Anguissola. Renaissance Woman, exhibition catalogue, S. Ferino-Pagden ed., Washington 1995

Washington 2009
The Art of Power. Royal Armor and Portraits from Imperial Spain, exhibition catalogue, A. Soler del Campo ed., Washington 2009

Washington and Los Angeles 1985
Collection for a King: Old Master Paintings from the Dulwich Picture Gallery, exhibition catalogue, G. Waterfield ed., Washington and Los Angeles 1985

Wellington 1901
E. Wellington, *A Descriptive & Historical Catalogue of the Collection of Pictures and Sculptures at Apsley House, London*, London 1901

Worcester 2005
Hope and Healing. Painting in Italy in a Time of Plague 1500–1800, exhibition catalogue, G.A. Bailey, P.M. Jones, F. Mormando and T.W. Worcester eds., Worcester 2005

Ximenez 1764
A. Ximenez, *Descripcion del Real Monasterio de San Lorenzo del Escorial*, Madrid 1764

Comparative Illustration Credits

Copyright credits:
fig. 1: Photograph © The State Hermitage Museum / photo by Vladimir Terebenin, Leonard Kheifets, Yuri Molodkovets
fig. 2: © Sovraintendenza di Roma Capitale – Foto in Comune
fig. 3: © Soprintendenza Speciale PS.A.E. e Polo Museale città di Firenze Gabinetto Fotografico
fig. 4: Image courtesy National Gallery of Art, Washington
fig. 5: © World rights
fig. 6: © The Trustees of the British Museum, London. All rights reserved
fig. 7: © The Trustees of the British Museum, London. All rights reserved
fig. 8: © The Trustees of the British Museum, London. All rights reserved
fig. 11: © Museo Interdisciplinare Regionale "A. Pepoli", Trapani
fig. 12: © Museo Nacional del Prado, Madrid
fig. 13: © The Trustees of the British Museum, London. All rights reserved.
fig. 14: © 2011. Photo Scala, Florence/Luciano Romano
fig. 16: © Patrimonio Nacional
fig. 21: © The Trustees of the British Museum, London. All rights reserved
fig. 22: © RMN / Droits réservés
fig. 28: Photograph © Bayerische Staatsgemäldesammlungen – Alte Pinakothek München
fig. 29: By kind permission of L'Assessorato per i Beni Culturali, Ambientali e P.I. della Regione siciliana. Dipartimento regionale dei Beni Culturali e Ambientali
fig. 35: © Kunsthistorisches Museum, Wien
fig. 36: Image © The Metropolitan Museum of Art
fig. 37: © Patrimonio Nacional
fig. 38: © By Permission of the Trustees of Dulwich Picture Gallery
fig. 41: By kind permission of l'Assessorato per i Beni Culturali e dell'Identità siciliana. Dipartimento Regionale BB. CC. e I.S.
fig. 42: Image © The Metropolitan Museum of Art

Photo credits:
pp. 12–13: © Xavier F. Salomon
fig. 9: © Xavier F. Salomon
fig. 10: © Xavier F. Salomon
fig. 11: Fotografia: Paolo Cracchiolo
fig. 15: Studio Elle Torino
fig. 18: © Xavier F. Salomon
fig. 19: © Xavier F. Salomon
fig. 20: © Xavier F. Salomon
fig. 24: © Xavier F. Salomon
fig. 27: Fotografia: Enzo Brai
fig. 31: © Xavier F. Salomon
fig. 32: Photograph Private Collection
fig. 34: © National Galleries of Scotland
fig. 41: Fotografia: Enzo Brai

Catalogue Entry Credits

Copyright credits:
cat 1: Image © The Metropolitan Museum of Art/Art Resource/Scala, Florence 2011
cat 2: © By Permission of the Trustees of Dulwich Picture Gallery
cat 3: © Patrimonio Nacional
cat 5: © The Trustees of the British Museum, London. All rights reserved
cat 9: © NTPL/John Hammond
cat 10: Houston Baptist University, Permanent Collection and gift from the Morris Collection Houston TX
cat 11: Museo Diocesano, Palermo
cat 13: © English Heritage Photo Library
cat 15: © Museo Nacional del Prado, Madrid
cat 16: Image © The Metropolitan Museum of Art/Art Resource/Scala, Florence 2011

Photo credits:
cat 1: © Photo Scala, Florence/The Metropolitan Museum of Art, 2011
cat 6: Matthew Hollow Photography
cat 14: Photo credit: Paul Hester
cat 16: © Photo Scala, Florence/The Metropolitan Museum of Art, 2011

Every attempt has been made to contact the copyright holders of these images. Unless stated above, all images supplied by the lender.

Silvana Editoriale Spa

via Margherita De Vizzi, 86
20092 Cinisello Balsamo, Milano
tel. 02 61 83 63 37
fax 02 61 72 464
www.silvanaeditoriale.it

Reproductions, printing and binding
by Arti Grafiche Amilcare Pizzi Spa
Cinisello Balsamo, Milan

Printed
January 2012